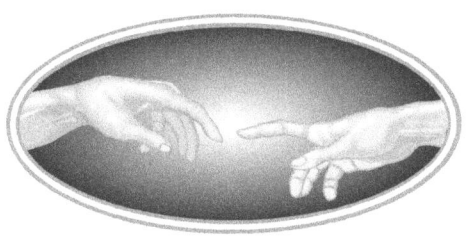

"Cancer Healing"

Live and Not Die

By: Richard K. McIlvaine

"Cancer Healing"

by: Richard K. McIlvaine

Copyrighted , All International Rights Reserved

ISBN-13: 978-1496152831
ISBN 10: 1496152832

Published by: Richard and Joy McIlvaine Publications
P.O. Box 315 – ISSAQUAH , WA USA 98027
Updated Version, New Title March, 2014

Email: RichardMcIlvaine@gmail.com

God's Words of Healing!

God wants to speak to you; listen to His Words:

"… I, the Lord, am your healer."
Exodus 15: 26

" I have heard your prayer,
I have seen your tears,
Behold,
I will heal you."
2 Kings 20: 5

"…forget none of His benefits:
Who pardons all your sins,
Who heals all your diseases…"
Psalm 103: 3

" He (Jesus) cast out spirits with a word,
and healed all who were ill
in order that what was spoken through
Isaiah the prophet might be fulfilled saying,
He Himself took our infirmities,
and carried away our diseases. "
Matthew 8: 16 – 18

Dedication

To Jesus
the One I love
A friend closer than a brother,
always True and Faithful,
the One who always comes through for me!
&
the Holy Spirit, the Helper and Comforter
the One who reveals these things!
&
My Father, the Heavenly Father, God, the One
whose lovingkindness
heard the cries of His children fighting against
Cancer
and sent His Word to heal them.

To Joy McIlvaine
My precious, loving wife,
and my children, Anna, John, and David

Table of Contents

God's Words of Healing

Table of Contents
Continued

Acknowledgments

We acknowledge that what is shared in this book came about by the mercy and grace of God sending forth the Holy Spirit to reveal keys to praying for the healing of cancer.

Also, we acknowledge God's intercessors and prophetic voices including Terry Reily, Walter Cowart, Welles & Katrin Hoffmann, Jerry & Penny Zelinsky, Gail Homan, Theresa Hammelman and family, Daniel Stevens, Corrine Gilmore, Keith & Debbie Webb, Greg & Mary Daley, John & Connye Scheda, Vivian Zoller, Ted & Lyn Allen, Cindy Manning, and Joy McIlvaine and others to numerous to name. Thank you for your prayers, encouragement and support in the unfolding of these keys that God's purposes and plans would be released.

We acknowledge all the Divine Healing Rooms Ministry Team, Advisors, and Intercessors in their faithful prayers and support during this time of seeking God for healing of those suffering from cancer.

Thank you to Nancy Crilly for stirring me on to finish this book and checking on its progress.

Also, thank you to my precious wife, Joy, who always inspires me with the love of God
flowing through her life to me and so many others to press on and complete this task.
Thank you to my three children Anna, John and David for supporting me in everything, in ministry and in the time taken to complete this book.

Acknowledgments
Continued

Thank you for my precious Aunt Marianne McIlvaine, a support through my whole life with God's ever faithful love and care. Thank you to a great supporter, Mrs. Barbara Cabot, a saint of God, whose support and trust during a difficult time inspired me to press through. It was through her battle with cancer many years ago that God spoke and confirmed some things revealed in this book. Thank you to Al & Mitzi Hametner for all their love, trust and support ! Thank you to Mitzi Hametner for your love, your fighting the good fight or faith, and all that we learned through your love, your prayers, and your battles.

Thank you to the precious Holy Spirit for coming and speaking the heart of God to bring healing to those suffering from cancer, answering the prayers of many for help.

Endorsements

"The Cancer Healing Rooms which provides prayer support for those fighting cancer is a welcome ministry being offered at the Divine Healing Rooms in the Seattle-Eastside.   Cancer is a word that many times paralyzes an individual with fear and despair. Rev. Rick and Joy McIlvaine who oversee the Cancer Healing Rooms are not intimidated by this word but are standing in faith with an anointing motivated by the love of God to see those battling cancer healed. The Holy Spirit has given Rick and Joy insights that I believe will be keys to help unlock the mystery that sometimes surrounds this disease. The gates of Hell shall not prevail and the Lord is raising people like the team at the Divine Healing Rooms who are willing to believe God for all his promises. They are knocking on the door of cancer and it shall not remain shut tight."

Rev. Greg J. Daley   August 2004
President, International Fellowship of Ministries (of John G. Lake heritage)
website: www.ifm7.org

"Reverend Richard and Joy McIlvaine have a deep desire to see people healed-body, soul and spirit. I have worked side by side with them and watched them diligently seek God for answers concerning healing. I believe God has given Richard and Joy revelation knowledge concerning healing of cancer as well as the gift of faith as they pray for individuals. Their teaching on healing builds faith for the non-believer as well as the mature believer to look to Jesus and receive their healing and salvation."

Fran L. Lance   Oct 14, 2004   Founder /Director Free Lance Ministries   www.franlance.org

Endorsements

Continued

"I commend this Cancer Healing Seminar to all those praying for their own healing or those praying for others with cancer. I gained great revelation of our authority over cancer and the practical application of that information on how to pray in faith. The revelation, taught with clarity and thoroughness, is based on and true to God's holy Word. God confirms his revelation by healing many through the prayer of faith combined with great anointing and gentle compassion. This seminar is a must."
Vivian Zoller, Intercessor, An Overcomer.   August 7, 2004

Introduction

We want to thank all the prayer warriors, intercessors and prophetic voices that have prayed over the last couple of years that God would speak to us and reveal "keys" to see cancer healed in the Divine Healing Rooms ministry. We want to acknowledge especially Brother Terry Reily and Rev.Walter Cowart of Seattle Revival Center, Newcastle, WA who both spoke to us and others of God's plans to release "keys" to seeing cancer healed in God's people.

Jesus said, "I will give you the keys of the kingdom of heaven; and whatever you bind on earth shall have been bound in heaven, and whatever you loose on earth shall have been loosed in heaven." Matthew 16:19

Jesus promised Peter and his disciples that He would give us "the keys to the Kingdom of Heaven". Keys are tools that unlock doors that otherwise would not be opened. We believe that today God's mercy and grace are coming to give us the "keys" we need to see cancer healed.

God's Word says in the Psalm 119:130 - "The unfolding of Your words gives light; It gives understanding to the simple." Over the last year and a half the Holy Spirit has been "unfolding" His Words to us and giving us understanding on how to see cancer healed.

Today we are still seeking Him for more understanding and trust God to continue revealing more "keys" to us to see even more people healed than we've seen already.

God is good, His mercies are new everyday and now we press on to believe that He will also reveal to us and others the "keys" to see Multiple Sclerosis, Parkinson's disease and other dreaded diseases healed on a consistent basis.

Preface

Be healed, be free of cancer, be restored and made whole in Jesus Name !
This is our prayer and hope for you in reading and utilizing the prayers, the declarations,
the Word of God and the information presented in this book.

For the next twenty-one days, the number of days seen in the Scriptures as the days needed for a breakthrough, I ask you to faithfully, daily, pray the prayers presented in this book and daily make the declarations stated.

In Daniel 10:13 we read, " But the prince of the kingdom of Persia was withstanding me for twenty-one days; then behold, Michael, one of the chief princes, came to help me, for I had been left there with the kings of Persia." Twenty-one days is the number of days for a breakthrough and this is the resistance time we need to break the "withstanding" of the cancer.

There are prayers for you to pray against the cancer in two different sections of this book and many proclamations listed for you to use. I recommend using these prayers two to three times a day at first until you begin to sense a change occurring, then you may want to reduce the amount of times. As you pray, be listening to the Holy Spirit to see if He would quicken to you any other Scriptures or prayers or ministry to bring healing to you.

The battle takes place on a couple of different fronts and each one is important.
On the one hand we need to receive mercy and healing and on the other hand do spiritual warfare. In this book we will present to you information on both. We have included also a list of recommended resources to help you receive your healing and be built up in your faith.

Preface
Continued

There is also the need, as you begin to pray and do spiritual battle, to allow the Holy Spirit to heal you body, soul, and spirit. The Holy Spirit wants to come in and heal the root sources of any hurts, sin or open doors to the enemy attacking you. Jesus said, " But when He, the Spirit of truth, comes, He will guide you into all the truth; for He will not speak on His own initiative, but whatever He hears, He will speak:" John 16:13

Each person is unique and our experience in ministering healing to those fighting cancer has taught us that we need to listen to the Holy Spirit in each instance. There is no intention in presenting this material to give you a "formula" for your healing. This book presents general information to give you help and insights into cancer to help you receive healing. There is no substitute for seeking the Lord to bring to you specific wisdom in your case to bring about your healing. Jeremiah 33:3 says, " Call to Me, and I will answer you, and tell you great and mighty things, which you do not know." Trust God to do that for you!

Forward

I recently read about the life of the famous inventor of the telegraph, Samuel F. B. Morse (1791-1872). In an interview, he was once asked,
"Professor Morse, when you were making your experiments at the university,
did you ever come to a standstill, not knowing what to do next?"

"I've never discussed this with anyone, so the public knows nothing about
it. But now that you ask me, I'll tell you frankly –
I prayed for more light."

"And did God give you the wisdom and knowledge you needed?"

"Yes, He did," said Morse. "That's why I never felt I deserved the honors
that came to me from America and Europe because of the invention associated
with my name. I had made a valuable application of the use of electrical
power, but it was all through God's help. It wasn't because I was superior
to other scientists. When the Lord wanted to bestow this gift on mankind,
He had to use someone. I'm just grateful He chose to reveal it to me."

In view of these facts, it's not surprising that the inventor's first message over the telegraph -- the very first transmitted message in history -- was: **"What hath God wrought!" Professor Morse must have had a
deeper revelation of what the Psalmist truly meant when he wrote,
"This is the Lord's doing"!**

Forward
Continued

We also acknowledge that the material in this book is the Lord's doing!

Our prayer has been and will be for God to send more light, more wisdom and knowledge
concerning the healing of cancer!

Glory to God !

Proclamations of Healing!

You must start changing what you say to receive what you believe and need!

Please read the following Scriptures to understand how powerful and important it is for you to proclaim what God says!

"Death and life are in the power of the tongue, and those who love it will eat its fruit."

Proverbs 18:21

Did you know there is "power" in your tongue! Power to speak "life" or "death"
Today begin to speak God's Words of "Life" not what you feel, not what the medical tests say, not your feelings, etc.

"With the heart man believes... with the mouth he confesses, resulting in salvation."
(salvation - saved from sickness and death) . Romans 10:10
Yes, we need to believe and "say" out loud God's words for the desired results of salvation!

"So faith comes by hearing, and hearing by the Word of Christ."
Romans 10:17
As you hear yourself speaking the Word of God, you will "hear" it and your faith will grow and grow like a mustard seed until it produces not just hope but real faith in your heart!

Please confess God's Words below out loud boldly. Say it over and over again until you believe it, until it moves from your head to your heart, faith will come, it will! Jesus said in Mark 11:22-23, "Have faith in God, Truly I say to you, whoever says to this mountain, 'Be taken up and cast into the sea,' and does not doubt in his heart, but believes that what he says is going to happen, it shall be granted him."

Proclamations of Healing!
Continued

"…Have mercy on us, Son of David!" Matthew 9:27

"I will not die, but live, and tell of the works of the Lord." Psalm 118:17

"He sent His Word and healed them and delivered them from their destructions." Psalm 107: 20

" The prayer offered in faith will restore the one who is sick, …" James 5: 15

"I have heard your prayer, I have seen your tears; behold, I will heal you."

Jeremiah 20:5

Let's begin by coming to God in prayer!

<u>Please pray and say out loud !!!</u>

<u>Jesus, "Son of David, Have mercy on me!"   Have mercy, Have mercy! Have mercy on me!</u>

Heavenly Father, I come to you now in the name of Jesus. I ask you to reveal yourself to me; I invite you to come into my life, my heart, my soul, and my body.

I give you permission to minister to me; I open my heart to you and cry out for your mercy and grace to come to me now.
I need you, I ask for your Holy Spirit to come to me now to reveal your love, your Presence and your healing power in my life.

You said in Your Word that "mercy triumphs over judgment", (James 2:13) so Father I ask You for Your Mercy to come now and remove by Your Great Mercy and Love any and all judgments in my life that may be enabling cancer in my body or keeping You from granting me repentance of any sin or healing and deliverance. Father, "deliver me from evil" !

I humbly come before you acknowledging that I have fallen short of your perfect will for my life and I ask you now to forgive me of my sins and to set me free from anything that would separate me from you.

I renounce anything and everything that is not pleasing to you God and ask you to reveal any such thing to me and set me free from it.

Coming to God in Prayer
Continued

I receive the precious blood of Jesus for the forgiveness of my sins and ask you, Jesus, to wash me with the water of your Word, renewing and regenerating me.

Jesus, you said that when the Holy Spirit comes that He would speak, that He would guide us into the truth and teach us all things. So I ask you now Holy Spirit to come and open up my mind to understand the things shared in the Word of God and in this book.

Heavenly Father, I ask you now in Jesus' Name to come and touch me, heal me, deliver me from this cancer, set me free from all sickness and affliction. I receive your mercy, your love, your forgiveness and your power and your healing in my body now. Thank you Father in Jesus Name!

In the name of Jesus, I break all the power of Satan to come and steal, kill, and destroy my life and command Satan and all his household and attacks to go from me now!

I ask you, Jesus, to come to me now and lead me into your perfect will, your abundant life!
Thank you Heavenly Father in Jesus Name'! Amen, Amen, and Amen!

(If you have not yet received Jesus as your personal Savior and experienced the words
of Jesus when He said, " you must be born again", please turn now to **Appendix A** in the back of this book in order to receive God's free gift of eternal life and enter into a new and living relationship with God.

Chapter 1

God speaks about Cancer!

God's Word!

"He sent His word and healed them, and delivered {them} from their destructions."

Psalm 107:20

Prayer Time!

Heavenly Father, I come to you in Jesus Name, like the blind man in the Bible.
I also cry out to you now, Son of David, (Jesus) have mercy on me! I ask you to forgive me of any sin in my life and I turn to you with all of my heart and ask you to come and reveal yourself to me now. I ask you to heal me from all cancer and restore me to perfect health. I ask you to open my mind to understand the Scriptures and to hear you speak to me. Thank you Father in Jesus' Name.

Proclaim over and over out loud!

"He Himself (Jesus) took our infirmities, and carried away our diseases."
(Jesus carried away your cancer, it was on Him
on the Cross !
What good news! – Believe that right now
and receive healing) Matthew 8:17

Chapter 1   God speaks about Cancer

Now is the time to let hope and faith rise up in your heart. God still heals today as He always has done and today is a good day for you to be healed and know the Love of God.

As you read the following pages, may the God of all Peace fill you with the knowledge of His Word and His will for you and bring healing and health to you.

"In the beginning God...." ; it always is that way and still today everything begins and ends with God speaking. His mercy comes to us and speaks words of life to us.

God started speaking to us about cancer out of the mouths of his intercessors and prophetic people. His servants began proclaiming that He was going to use the Divine Healing Rooms – Seattle Eastside and the Seattle Revival Center, an Assembly of God church in Newcastle, WA, as a place of healing for cancer.

Wow! These were unusual, startling words for one to hear and we did not know at the time what to make of it. This took place in the beginning of the year 2002. As time went on we would occasionally hear God speak these same words again, but over a year of silence went by before the first revelation knowledge about cancer began to come.

Chapter 1   God speaks about Cancer

Psalm 119:130 says, "The unfolding of Thy words gives light; It gives understanding to the simple." This is exactly what began to take place. God began unfolding His Words like pieces of a puzzle that we had to pray and ask Him about to understand. Today we continue seeking Him and asking Him for more knowledge and understanding.

God said in Isaiah 55: 8-9, " For My thoughts are not your thoughts, neither are your ways My ways, declares the Lord. For as the heavens are higher than the earth, So are My ways higher than your ways. And My thoughts than your thoughts." So, as the Holy Spirit impressed God's thoughts in my heart I lifted them back up to Him for understanding.
As time went on, God gave more! The process was like "pieces of a puzzle" coming together!

What we are about to share with you is what we call "revelation" knowledge. It is not the repeating of something learned, taught or read some place. Jesus said, "Blessed are you Simon Barjona, because flesh and blood did not reveal this to you, but my Father who is in heaven."
Matthew 16:18. Today we believe the Father is still revealing things that flesh and blood, the human mind, would never be able to figure out.

It began without any notice. The Holy Spirit impressed these awesome words in my heart in the beginning of 2003;

"Cancer is human cells taking on a life of their own."

Chapter 1   God speaks about Cancer
_____

What awesome words, words revealing how God views cancer from the heavenly realm of "His thoughts". I began to chew and meditate on these words to try to understand what God was saying about cancer by these words.

Hearing God speak about cancer is really exciting to me because I believe He would only be speaking about it in order to reveal how to be healed of this dreaded disease.

So, what did God mean by "cancer is human cells taking on a life of their own" ? I asked over and over again trying to grasp how this could be used to minister healing to those suffering from cancer. I asked questions such as, "How can we get these cells to stop taking on a life of their own and similar?

Later I heard the Holy Spirit speak more to me. These words were very shocking to me!

" How can you get mad at your cells for taking on a life of their own when you are doing the same thing in your own heart?"

Wow! Now we have a connection between what is happening in the body, cancer, and what's happening in the heart.

The Holy Spirit continued on,

"Ever since Eve, man has been taking on a life of his own and the sin has been piling up and piling up, and cancer more and more will build up."

Chapter 1   God speaks about Cancer

The above reference to "Eve" would seem to relate to Eve choosing to turn aside from God's will for her in the garden of Eden to eat of the "Tree of Life" to the eating of the forbidden "Tree of the knowledge of Good & Evil".

So, from all these words I began to seek to understand how what was happening in the heart of man was tied together with what was happening in the cells of the body.

God reveals things to us by the very words He uses. He uses the words "cancer is the human cells taking on a life of their own" not to confound us but to give us understanding of what is going on here. He wants us to search out the meaning and the very process of that gives us understanding we could not otherwise grasp.

We see here God revealing that cancer starts at the human cell level.

In looking up the definition of the word "cancer" on the Internet I found this quote,

"What is cancer? In the simplest terms, cancer is a disease initiated by your own body, where **your own cells** start to proliferate madly and uncontrollably, until these cancer cells disrupt normal systems and eventually kill the body. If you think about it, it's kind of like unintentional suicide."

Off Internet Search - Health Correspondent- "Every 2nd Saturday", August 6, 2004

Chapter 1   God speaks about Cancer

One of the confirmations I received of this understanding of cancer being something rooted within 'us' was from a newspaper article. The timing of this was just the next day after really seeking God about cancer being related to us primarily, our heart, and not mostly some outside causes or substances. Let me say though, that I do believe that other things can cause cancer too.

On the morning of August 4, 2004, I opened the front page section of The Seattle Times newspaper sitting in front of me to the middle for some reason and lo and behold I had opened the paper to a full page article headline titled, " Cancer, the Incurable?". I was surprised that they would put this article in the front section of the paper and not the "B" or "C" section where articles like this usually occur.

As I quickly glanced over the full page article a man's picture and quote caught my eye and I read the following words of Dr. Craig Henderson, Breast-cancer specialist, University of California, San Francisco, and President of Access Oncology, a drug developer; "What we have learned by these billions of dollars invested in cancer biology is that **cancers are us** …Identify what makes cancer unique and wipe it out? That won't happen. We cannot wipe out the cancer without wiping out a lot of the rest of us."
Seattle Times, page A-3, August 4, 2003

Our cells are not supposed to "take on a life of their own". They were created to serve and support "our life", not to create another life within our bodies. Yet this is what is taking place.

As the cells do that they seek to "use our life", "our body" as their support system to grow and live off us much like a parasite would do to its host. This is contrary to the divine order of God's plan for our cells and body.

Chapter 1   God speaks about Cancer

These cells have become renegade cells, lawless, rebellious, out of control and contrary to their original God given and genetic design. To stop this process, to heal cancer we must go to the source, the root of what enables and empowers these cells to do such a thing.

God saying, "How can you get mad at your cells for taking on a life of their own when you are doing the same thing in your own heart?", ties together what is happening in the cells (going their own way, acting lawless, growing out of control) to a similar situation in our own heart.   He is saying that we have been doing the same thing our cells are doing by "taking on a life of our own" in our hearts, in our lives. So, how can be we be mad if our cells have decided to do the same thing?

God sees this "taking on a life of their own" as a sin against Him as evidenced by His very next words after that: "Ever since Eve, man has been taking on a life of his own and the sin has been piling up and piling up, and cancer more and more will build up." Not only is it sin but this sin has continued down from generation to generation since Adam and Eve until now it seems to have reached some sort of "critical mass" whereby cancer will "build up" or increase more and more in people.

This agrees with what we read in the Scriptures concerning what we call generational sin. God's Word in Exodus 34:7 says, "…who keeps lovingkindness for thousands, who forgives iniquity, transgression and sin; yet He will by no means leave {the guilty} unpunished, visiting the iniquity of fathers on the children and on the grandchildren to the third and fourth generations."

Also, we see sin from the time of Adam & Eve affecting all of us in the Scripture found in Romans 5:12; " Therefore, just as through one man sin entered into the world, and death through sin, and so death spread to all men, because all sinned -…"

(See Appendix B – Scriptures relating to Generational curses for more study on this subject.)

So, putting all of this together we begin to see a picture of what happens in our heart affecting not just the heart or soul of a man but also affecting the physical cells of the body.

God's words seem to indicate a direct connection between cancer in the cells and what's happening in the heart (the soul – the mind, will and emotions). So as the heart goes so the human cells go. Our hearts "taking on a life of our own" seems to be a sin allowing our cells also to "take on a life of their own". This only compounds as it continues from generation to generation, being passed down in the lives of our children.

Most of us are aware of this principle of the effects of stress in our physical bodies from our own experiences or from hearing about it on television programs. If we allow stress in our bodies over a period of time it ends up causing stomach ulcers, hives, shingles, rashes, heart problems and the list goes on and on. Stress is in our "soul," yet it works outwardly to eventually affect our physical body with symptoms of sickness.

Chapter 1   God speaks about Cancer

Let's look at some Scriptures from God's Word that speak about these things:

"The heart is more deceitful than all else and is desperately sick; Who can understand it?"   Jeremiah 17:9

"All of us like sheep have gone astray, Each of us has turned to his own way; But the LORD has caused the iniquity of us all to fall on Him."   Isaiah 53:6

"But you said in your heart, 'I will ascend to heaven; I will raise my throne above the stars of God, and I will sit on the mount of assembly in the recesses of the north.
'I will ascend above the heights of the clouds; I will make myself like the Most High.'
Nevertheless you will be thrust down to Sheol, to the recesses of the pit."   Isaiah 14:13-15

"Open shame belongs to us, O Lord, to our kings, our princes and our fathers, because we have sinned against You. To the Lord our God {belong} compassion and forgiveness, for we have rebelled against Him; nor have we obeyed the voice of the LORD our God, to walk in His teachings which He set before us through His servants the prophets.
Indeed all Israel has transgressed Your law and turned aside, not obeying Your voice; so the curse has been poured out on us, along with the oath which is written in the law of Moses the servant of God, for we have sinned against Him." Daniel 9: 8-11

Chapter 1   God speaks about Cancer

"Before I was afflicted I went astray, But now I keep Your
word."

Psalm 119:67

"Do not be wise in your own eyes; Fear the LORD and turn
away from evil.
It will be healing to your body and refreshment to your bones."

Proverbs 3:7,8

"as it is written, "THERE IS NONE RIGHTEOUS, NOT
EVEN ONE;
THERE IS NONE WHO UNDERSTANDS, THERE IS
NONE WHO SEEKS FOR GOD;
ALL HAVE TURNED ASIDE, ..."

Romans 3:10-12

Jesus said, ""Behold, you have become well; do not sin
anymore, so that nothing worse happens to you."

John 5: 14

Chapter 1   God speaks about Cancer

(See Appendix C – More Scriptures relating Sin &
Sickness
sometimes tied together !)

In the following chapter we will look to further define what sin " taking on a life of our own" is so that we can more clearly deal with it.

Chapter 2

The spiritual Root Cause of Cancer!

God's Word!

"For whoever wishes to save his life will lose it, but whoever loses his life for My sake and the gospel's will save it." Mark 8:35

Prayer Time!

Heavenly Father, I come to you in Jesus Name, I invite your Holy Spirit to come and minister to me and to show me anything in my heart that is not pleasing to you. I ask you to speak to me personally as I read these pages and to bring revelation knowledge to me for my own life and for others. Thank you Father in Jesus Name.

Proclaim Over and Over out Loud!

"...for by His (Jesus') wounds you were healed."

2 Peter 2:25

Chapter 2   The spiritual Root Cause of Cancer!

God wants to heal you all the way down to the root cause of cancer so that it won't keep coming back again and again. We are looking for a "cure", not to just keep dealing with reoccurring symptoms of a root cause.

Just like dandelions in your yard, if you just cut off the top part that you can see and don't remove the root you can't see, the dandelion will grow back again later. We need to find and remove the root of cancer so it can't keep growing back. That root cause God is revealing does not start in the body but in the heart, so we must go to the heart first to find a cure.

While I was praying and seeking the Lord specifically about what sin "taking on a life of our own" was to Him, He continued to bring revelation.

As I was typing the beginning insights the Lord had shared with me to send out in an email prayer for someone with cancer, I unexpectedly heard the Holy Spirit speak to me and say, " Romans 6 ".

The Holy Spirit began speaking "rhema" (the Greek word for 'breath') words (words that are quickened to your spirit as if God were speaking them personally only to you) to me as I read Romans 6 starting in verse 12.

Romans 6:12 says, " Therefore do not let sin reign in your mortal body that you should obey its lusts, …" This scripture reveals to us that sin and our "mortal bodies" effect each other.

Chapter 2   The spiritual Root Cause of Cancer!

As I continued reading, the Holy Spirit continued to quicken and speak to me through the Scriptures in Romans 6 from verses 12 all the way to the end of the chapter in verse 23.

When I got down to Romans 6:19 and was reading, " I am speaking in human terms because of the weakness of your flesh. <u>For just as you presented your members as slaves to impurity and to lawlessness, resulting in {further} lawlessness,</u> so now present your members as slaves to righteousness, resulting in sanctification."

At the point of reading the words, " resulting in further lawlessness", I unexpectedly heard the Holy Spirit plainly speak to me saying, "<u>That is Cancer</u>"! Wow! I was surprised!

I have read that verse many times before and sometimes wondered what that "resulting in further lawlessness" part meant. I believe the Holy Spirit is revealing through His words that lawlessness in our life breeds the further lawlessness of the cells in our body to now also become lawless, to grow out of control, to "take on a life of their own"- thus Cancer!

Lawlessness is defined as the "rejection of the law, or will, of God and the substitution of the will of self ". Vines Expository Dictionary of New Testament words, page 657.

(<u>See Appendix "E" – All verses of Romans 6: 12-23 relating to lawlessness,</u>
<u>"resulting in further lawlessness" – Cancer !</u>)

Chapter 2   The spiritual Root Cause of Cancer!

To more clearly understand the spiritual root of cancer I took all these things He was saying back to God in prayer. I was seeking a concise answer, something simple, something that made sense to me, to everyone. I believed that in the end the answer would be as God says in His Word, "But the wisdom from above is first pure, then peaceable, gentle, reasonable, full of mercy and good fruits, unwavering, without hypocrisy." James 3:17

As I sought the Lord I took to Him what I had received, "human cells taking on a life of their own", "the same thing in your own heart", and "the sin has been piling up" and asked to hear from Him what He would say is the spiritual root of cancer. I didn't want to figure it out in my own mind and miss it.

The answer came in a vision from God. He used what He had taught me in the past, what I knew, to reveal to me what I did not know.   In this vision I saw a picture of the ends of two bones hanging in mid air. He began speaking about how in the past He had used an illustration of the joints between bones to teach me about the spiritual root cause of arthritis in some cases. He revealed then that arthritis was pain between the bones in the joints and that the pain between the bones was a spiritual reflection of the pain between two people in the Body of Christ.

The Scriptures use bones to speak of parts of the Body of Christ being joined together into a dwelling place of God in the Spirit. (Ephesians 4:16)

Chapter 2 _____ The spiritual Root Cause of Cancer!

The pain between the two parts of the Body of Christ was the sin of unforgiveness. The spiritual root sin of unforgiveness was reflected in the physical body in a corresponding way. Something between people (i.e. pain, an irritation, no love between them) was now manifesting itself in a similar way in the natural, physical realm - pain in the joints.

I remembered how many, many years ago I had prayed for a woman over eighty years old who was a friend of my mother's friend. She walked into the house we were visiting with a cane in hand and moved very slowly, tiny step by tiny step. Later I asked if I could pray for her. She said she had arthritis real bad and that it was very painful in her knees. While praying I heard the Holy Spirit say, "Tell her to forgive her mother and she will be healed." I asked her if this was true about her mother? She said "Yes" it was true! Then I asked her if she would forgive her mother for the hurts and she said that she would. Afterwards when I went to pray against the arthritis in her knees the power of God hit her and she jumped up and began walking then running around the room without her cane. Years later I checked up on her through my Mom and found out she was still walking around without a cane and doing very well. Praise God!

James 5:16 says, "Therefore, confess your sins to one another, and pray for one another so that you may be healed." Many times sin and sickness are tied together but I don't believe the Scriptures teach that is the case in all situations. We need to listen to the Holy Spirit each time for each person and see what He says; it may vary from person to person.

Chapter 2   The spiritual Root Cause of Cancer!

Going back to the vision of the bones and God using what I had learned in the past to teach me today what I don't know; God then took me to a comparison of the "pain between the bones" being arthritis from the sin of unforgiveness to "cells taking on a life of their own," lawlessness being cancer from the spiritual root sin of _____?

I still didn't try to say what it was; I just listened. I wanted to hear God say what it would be not me. As I waited, I heard the Holy Spirit say to me, "the sin of pride". Wow! There it was! The spiritual root of cancer!

Wow! Pride! Let me think! Pride- what is that? I began to use my mind to compare "pride" to "human cells taking on a life of their own", "lawlessness", "ever since Eve", "doing the same thing in your heart", and the words of Dr. Craig Henderson, the cancer specialist, " cancer is us".

What is pride? I thought of the Scriptures we call the "Five I wills"; an allegory where speaking of Satan it says, "But you said in your heart, 'I will ascend to heaven; I will raise my throne above the stars of God, And I will sit on the mount of assembly In the recesses of the north. 'I will ascend above the heights of the clouds; I will make myself like the Most High.'
"Nevertheless you will be thrust down to Sheol, To the recesses of the pit." Isaiah 14:13-15

Pride was the first sin! Satan said "in his heart" – I will! He got his eyes off God and put them on himself and turned aside from God's Will to pursue "his own will".

Chapter 2   The spiritual Root Cause of Cancer!

Satan pursuing his "own will" is the sin that got him thrown out of Heaven to the earth where he immediately began to deceive man into doing the same thing.

He convinced Eve in the garden to commit the same sin. Satan deceived her and she turned aside from "God's will" to eat from the "Tree of Life" and ate from the forbidden "Tree of the knowledge of Good & Evil". She took on a "life of her own" outside of God's plan.

Listen to the words of Isaiah the prophet, " All of us like sheep have gone astray, Each of us has turned to his own way;..." Isaiah 53:6

Cancer is human cells "gone astray", "turned to their own way", taking on a "will of their own", lawless, no longer following the divine plan. In essence our cells begin to say, " I will", "I will", "I will" and "take on a life of their own" regardless of the genetic, God ordained plan for them. They keep growing and growing lawlessly out of order to create their own life outside of the body's life ultimately killing its host, our body.

The type of pride, as there are different types of pride, that is the spiritual root of cancer is what I would call "self determination pride". This helps bring an understanding of the type of pride we are dealing with here. When most people think of "pride" they only think of the kind that shows itself when someone is arrogant, proud, and looks at themselves in the mirror a lot.

Chapter 2   The spiritual Root Cause of Cancer!

As I sought to understand this **"sin of pride"** and what form it took, I believe the Holy Spirit took me to some Scriptures to clearly see an example of how this looks.

Listen to these words, "Come now, you who say, "Today or tomorrow we will go to such and such a city, and spend a year there and engage in business and make a profit.

Yet you do not know what your life will be like tomorrow. You are {just} a vapor that appears for a little while and then vanishes away.

Instead, {you ought} to say, "If the Lord wills, we will live and also do this or that."

But as it is, you boast in your arrogance; all such boasting is evil."   James 4:13-16

God's Word in 1 John seems to relate to the same type of pride;
"For all that is in the world, the lust of the flesh and the lust of the eyes and the boastful pride of life, is not from the Father, but is from the world.

The world is passing away, and {also} its lusts; but the one who does the will of God lives forever."   1 John 2:16,17

Jesus said, "For from within, out of the heart of men, proceed the evil thoughts, fornications, thefts, murders, adulteries, deeds of coveting {and} wickedness, {as well} {as} deceit, sensuality, envy, slander, pride {and} foolishness.

All these evil things proceed from within and defile the man."
                                            Mark 7: 21-23

Chapter 2   The spiritual Root Cause of Cancer!

This type of pride seems to be the "kind" that always exposes itself " in spoken words". Satan said, " I will" five times! In James 4:13 we see "you who say, "Today or tomorrow, we will"". This is all about "whose" will is going to be in control.

In cancer, the human cells have taken control, they seek to exert their own will over the body's plan to create cells that live and die in just the right pattern to support the life of the body.
These cells have taken on "a life of their own" and have no regard for the "life of the body" or how their "doings" will affect any other cells or organs or systems in the body.

Typically this type of pride that is the spiritual root of cancer discloses itself with words spoken such as these: "I will", " That will never happen to me", "I am going to have this and that and do this and live there", "I'm never going to be like that", "I am never going to be poor",
"I am never going to get cancer like that person", and these types of sayings.

One of the things the Lord used to confirm this to me was the bringing back to my mind
of an incident that occurred many years before. Interestingly enough it happened while praying for a dear saint of God in the hospital fighting cancer with doctors only giving her a very short time to live. While praying for her the Holy Spirit said, "she has sinned". I could hardly believe this dear woman had a single sin. I asked the Holy Spirit to reveal the sin. He said "the sin of pride".

Chapter 2   The spiritual Root Cause of Cancer!

This woman seemed to be the most humble Christian I knew and I was really struggling sharing this with her but I did anyway. As I shared with her she came under conviction of the Holy Spirit and asked God to forgive her with tears. I asked her what sin of pride she had committed. She shared a story about a time in her life years before when standing in line at a store she overheard a woman in front of her lamenting to the clerk about her battle with cancer. She went on to say that when she heard that she said to herself, " That will never happen to me, I won't ever get cancer." I have always remembered this because it was so unusual in that she seemed to so quickly know how she had committed that sin and so vividly remembered it.

Since this time it has been amazing to me to listen to people's conversations to see how often we say these types of things in normal everyday conversation; it has been a little shocking to me. Scripture says in Hosea 4:6, "My people are destroyed for lack of knowledge."

We need the knowledge of the Word of God and the ministry of the Holy Spirit not to sin against God.

Praise God for Jesus, that He came to set us free from sin. Jesus said, "… and you will know the truth, and the truth will make you free." John 8: 32 and also, "If therefore the Son shall make you free, you shall be free indeed." John 8:36

There is good news; God tells us, "If we confess our sins, He is faithful and righteous to forgive us our sins and to cleanse us from all unrighteousness. If we say that we have not sinned, we make Him a liar and His word is not in us. My little children, I am writing these things to you so that you may not sin. And if anyone sins, we have an Advocate with the Father, Jesus Christ the righteous;" 1 John 1:9,10; 2:1

Chapter 3

Removing the authority of Cancer

God's Word!

"Fear the Lord and turn away from evil. It will be healing to your body, and refreshment to your bones."
Proverbs 3: 7,8

Prayer Time!

Heavenly Father, I come to you in Jesus' Name; Have mercy on me! Forgive me of my sins, wash me in the blood of Jesus. Wash me with the water of your Word, renewing and regenerating me that I might know you. Heal me, deliver me from this evil of cancer. Set me free from the power of Satan. Jesus come into my life, my heart, my body and restore me, make me whole. I want you and need you and ask you to reveal your plans, your will and destiny for my life.
Thank you Father in Jesus Name.

Proclaim over and over out Loud!

"...and the prayer offered in faith will restore the one who is sick,..." James 5:15

Chapter 3   Removing the authority of Cancer

How do we stop cancer? How can we stop these cells from multiplying? How can we keep it from coming back over and over again?

We must remove the root cause of the cancer. We must get at and remove the spiritual root of the cancer so that it can no longer come back. In the previous chapter we discovered that spiritual root to be "the sin of pride", the self-determination type of pride that seeks to ignore God's Will and seek after its own will in a selfish, ambitious sort of way. Remember also that this is a generational sin with the sin being passed down from generation to generation. The generational sin must also be dealt with through the remitting of the sins of the forefathers.

One of the things the Holy Spirit said about cancer was: **" How can you get mad at your cells for taking on a life of their own when you are doing the same thing in your own heart?"**

Removing cancer starts in the heart! That "doing the same thing in your own heart" has to be stopped because that's where the human cells are gaining the right, authority and power to rebel, act lawlessly, and to "take on a life of their own".

Jesus said, "For from within, out of the heart of men, proceed... deceit, sensuality, envy, slander, pride {and} foolishness." Mark 7: 21,22

First things first! Where do we start? We start freedom from cancer by coming to God and crying out, crying out and crying out for **HIS MERCY to come and remove the judgment of cancer caused by generations of sin and my own sins**. **"Son of David, Have mercy on me"!**
Go ahead, keep crying out for His Mercy over and over again until there is no more breath in you or you have the assurance in your heart of having received it!

God's Word says, " ...Mercy triumphs over judgment."
James 2:13

We need God's mercy to come and remove any and all judgments against past generations and me so that I can repent, so that I can receive healing and deliverance. Healing and deliverance Scriptures and quoting the Word will not remove judgments that have come because of the unrepentant sin of pride and lawlessness, etc. "Mercy" is God's provision to remove any judgments. Judgments can be operating in our life and we are not even aware of it and yet just the same it is still hindering us from receiving the ability to repent, healing or deliverance.

Judgment is something we don't want to think about- it is kind of scary, it sounds bad. Yet God have provided a remedy for it when it occurs. It is not the end of the world. God's mercy in many instances in the Bible came to remove judgments in people's lives because of sin.

"For he who eats and drinks, eats and drinks <u>judgment to himself,</u> if he does not <u>judge the body rightly.</u> (repent, stop doing wrong) For this reason many among you are weak and sick, and a number sleep (die). But <u>if we judged ourselves rightly, we should not be judged.</u> (our goal) But when we are judged, we are disciplined by the Lord in order that we may NOT be condemned along with the world."   1 Corinthians 11: 29-32

"Therefore, let us draw near with confidence to the Throne of Grace, so that we may <u>receive mercy</u> and find grace to help in time of need." (the need of healing) Hebrews 4:16

Receive God's mercy now, the blood of Jesus was shed that we might receive God's mercy and not under any past or present judgments. With judgment out of the way, we can move on to: the receiving of forgiveness of our sins; the sins of past generations in our family; the entering into of true repentance of the sin of "I will" - self-determination pride with the fruit of it showing; and lastly the receiving of healing and deliverance of the cancer. This can all happen quickly, within moments of coming to God, it doesn't have to take long, it's a matter of the heart.

After asking God for mercy, the healing of cancer continues in the heart! We begin by allowing the Holy Spirit to show us our sin; asking Him to show us our heart and any "I will" pride that may be lurking in there that needs to be rooted out. This "I will" pride is seen most easily by watching the words we say. It comes out by us saying things that seem to say we can control the outcome of our lives as if we were God. It comes out as us seeking to control others, the outcome of other people's lives, the outcome of events, situations, etc. as if we were in control and not God. It comes out as: "I want" "I will never" "that will never happen" ,etc.

Chapter 3   Removing the authority of Cancer

1 Corinthians 11: 28 instructs us, " But let a man examine himself, …" As we examine ourselves, the Holy Spirit will help us and reveal any sin or pride within our heart.

As we "see our sin" and allow godly sorrow of that which hurts God to arise in our heart, we, by the grace of God, can choose to turn away from it, or what we call repent from it and renounce it in our lives. Then we need to ask God to forgive us of this sin of pride and wash us in the precious blood of Jesus to thoroughly remove its stain.

Next we need to ask Jesus to wash us with the "water of the Word" to change our hearts, renew our hearts, and regenerate our hearts that we might not sin against Him anymore in this area.

We see this powerful effect of Jesus washing us in Ephesians 5:26,27 " that He might sanctify her, having cleansed her by the washing of water with the Word, that He might present to Himself the church in all her glory, having no spot or wrinkle or any such thing; but that she should be holy and blameless."

"For thus the Lord GOD, the Holy One of Israel, has said, 'In repentance and rest you will be saved,' … Isaiah 30:15

This repentance of sin, this turning away from the sin of self-determination pride and the submitting to God's will instead of our will, is a key in being healed of cancer.

This forgiveness of our sin and the remitting of the generational sins of our forefathers brings us into a legal position on earth in the Kingdom of God to gain the authority and right to "deal with" human cells acting lawlessly.

In the Scriptures below we see an illustration of how important authority is in dealing with spiritual matters and in healing.

"Now Jesus {started} on His way with them; and when He was not far from the house, the centurion sent friends, saying to Him, "Lord, do not trouble Yourself further, for I am not worthy for You to come under my roof;
for this reason I did not even consider myself worthy to come to You, but {just} say the word, and my servant will be healed.
For I also am a man placed under authority, with soldiers under me; and I say to this one, 'Go!' and he goes, and to another, 'Come!' and he comes, and to my slave, 'Do this!' and he does it."
Now when Jesus heard this, He marveled at him, and turned and said to the crowd that was following Him, "I say to you, not even in Israel have I found such great faith." Luke 7: 7-9

The centurion soldier said to Jesus, "I too, am a man under authority, with soldiers under me; and I say to this one, 'Go!' and he goes;

This soldier understood that being "under authority" was the key to "having authority".
In that place he was able to exert authority and say, 'Go!' and he goes;…"

This is the kind of authority necessary to say to the cancerous cells, 'Go!' and they go. We are seeking after the kind of authority that gives us the legal right to speak to God created cells, human living cells that God called 'good'.

As we remove in our heart the lawlessness and stop taking on a "life of our own" we come "under authority", "under God's authority", and having submitted to God, we now gain the authority and the right to command the cancerous human cells to also no longer "take on a life of their own".

Something else I heard the Holy Spirit speak to me during all this was a Scripture out of the book of James.

James 4:7,8 says, " Submit therefore to God. Resist the devil and he will flee from you."

As I read those words I heard the Spirit of God speak to me and say, "Submit to God and resist cancer and it will flee from you, Submit to God and resist anything not of God and it will flee from you."

Authority and power, the right to "Resist the devil" and see him flee came out of
first 'Submitting to God'. As we first submit to God we can exercise power and authority to resist cancer cells and see them flee!

We also see this principle in Proverbs 3:7,8, "Fear the Lord and turn away from evil. It will be healing to your body and refreshment to your bones."

Chapter 3   Removing the authority of Cancer

Here we see a clear example of how turning away from evil brings healing to the physical body. The "turn from evil" takes place in the heart releasing healing in the body.

Another Scripture that reveals a connection between what the heart does and the body is found in Psalm 119: 67,68; "Before I was afflicted I went astray, But now I keep Your word.
You are good and do good; Teach me Your statutes."

We would like to think that there are no consequences to going astray from God's Word but God's Word instructs us differently. This gaining of the ability and authority to deal with physical sickness by actions in the soul realm is also seen in James 5: 16: "Therefore, confess your sins to one another, and pray for one another so that you may be healed. The effective prayer of a righteous man can accomplish much."

I want to ask you at this point to do something very difficult if you truly sincerely are willing to do everything and anything to be healed of cancer.

Would you be willing to ask your wife or husband, a family member, a close friend who knows you well, who practically lives with you daily, to lovingly share with you every time you speak or do something that is an expression of: "I will", "self-will determination" , controlling the outcome of themselves or others or situations? Would you create a spiritual atmosphere that fosters this kind of accountability with this person? Would you not get mad at them, attack them, retaliate against them, distance yourself from them, etc. until the fruits of repentance that John the Baptist called for are manifested in their life. Go ahead, do it now with that person!

Chapter 4

Prayer for Healing of Cancer - Part 1

God's Word!

"… and the prayer offered in faith will restore the one who
is sick, and the Lord will raise him up, and if he has
committed sins, they will be forgiven him."
James 5:15

Proclaim Over and Over out Loud !

"I will not die, but live, and tell of the works of the Lord.
The Lord has disciplined me severely, But He has not
given me over to death."
Psalm 118:17,18

Prayer for Healing of Cancer- Part 1
Prayer of forgiveness, repentance and renouncing !

Please pray with me now! Lay one hand on your area of cancer
or on your head and the other towards Heaven. Pray with me from
your heart and out loud looking to the mercy
and grace of God to heal you! Look to Jesus and don't look for any
feelings, just simply believe.

Heavenly Father, God of Abraham, Isaac, and Jacob, I come to
you, the One true God, in the Name of Your Son Jesus. I believe
Jesus that you died for me, that you rose again, that you took my sins
and my sicknesses and pains on the cross and I praise and thank you
now for your great salvation. I ask you for mercy, have mercy on
me; remove any judgments of sin from me and my past generations.

Chapter 4   Prayer for Healing of Cancer - Part 1

Heavenly Father, my body, my cells have gone their own way, they have taken on a life of their own, they have gone astray, they are going their own way, they are no longer following the divine pattern of life you created.

We all have gone astray like sheep your Word says. I confess Father in Jesus Name
my sin. I have gone astray, my past family generations also have gone astray. We have not followed you, your divine will, and your divine life for us; we have strayed away many times and in many ways. We have committed the sin of pride; we have said in our own hearts that
"I will", "I will", "I will" many, many times and have taken on our own life, gone our own way over and over and over again.

Forgive me Father of my sin, forgive me of pride, of going my own way, of going astray from "Your life" to take on a life of my own. I am sorry, I repent, and I ask you to forgive me, forgive my past family generations going back all the way to Adam and Eve of the sin of pride.

Chapter 4   Prayer for Healing of Cancer - Part 1

I remit their sins to you and ask you to wash my forefathers and me in the blood of Jesus and cleanse us.

I renounce in Jesus Name all pride, all taking on of my own life, of going my own way.
I repent, I turn to you Father in Jesus Name and by your grace and help, I now declare that I will "Follow Jesus", I will do what Jesus said in His Word in John 21:22. I will obey Romans 12:1,2.

I renounce my heart, my soul, my life taking on its own life and I give my life to you as a living sacrifice and I turn to only follow you, to ask you, to seek you, to listen and obey you from this point on, in Jesus Name. Amen.

Now in the Name of Jesus, I command every cell in my body to STOP taking on a life of its own. My heart and life is no longer "taking on a life of its own" and now in the Name of Jesus Christ I rebuke you cancer cells and command you now to no longer take on a life of your own!!!

Now in the Name of Jesus I command every cell in my body to come back into divine order. In the Name of Jesus I rebuke every cancerous cell now in my body and command it to die, shrink up, dissolve, dissipate, leave, go, be removed from my body and never return.

Chapter 4   Prayer for Healing of Cancer - Part 1

Heavenly Father in Jesus Name I now receive my healing from Jesus, I receive your mercy and grace and healing anointing in my body. Heal me, make me whole! I receive healing to any and all damage done to my body by the cancer, for by His stripes we were healed.

I ask you to bring life to my body, to strengthen me, I need your help, and I receive your encouragement, your power, and your life in me now at this moment.

Thank you Father in Jesus Name!! Amen, Amen and Amen.

Thank you for Your Word, "By His stripes we were healed". 1 Peter 2:24

Thank you for Your Word, "No weapon formed against me shall prosper." Isaiah 54:17

Thank you for Your Word, "HE HIMSELF TOOK OUR INFIRMITIES AND CARRIED
AWAY OUR DISEASES." Matthew 8:17

Thank you for Your Word, "I will not die, but live, and tell of the works of the Lord."

Psalm 118:17
Thank you for Your Word, "Who heals all your diseases; …"
Psalm 103: 3

Thank you for Your Word, "I will rescue him, and honor him, with long life I will satisfy
him, and let him behold My salvation." Psalm 91: 15,16

Thank you for Your Word, "I cried to Thee for help, and Thou didst heal me." Psalm 30:2

Chapter 5

Breaking the Power Of the spirit of Cancer !

God's Word!

" Thus says the Lord, the God of your father David, 'I have heard your prayer, I have seen your tears; behold, I will heal you. On the third day you shall go up to the house of the Lord."   2 Kings 20:5

Prayer Time

Heavenly Father, I ask you to set me free from any attacks of the enemy. Your Word says Satan comes to steal, kill, and destroy but Jesus came to give life and give it abundantly. I receive that abundant life now.
Thank you Father in Jesus Name.

Proclaim Over and Over out Loud!

"Beloved, I pray that in all respects you may prosper and be in good health,
just as your soul prospers." 3 John 2

Chapter 5   Breaking the power of the spirit of Cancer

God's Word says, "For our struggle is not against flesh and blood, but against the rulers, against the powers, against the world forces of this darkness, against the spiritual {forces} of wickedness in the heavenly {places.} Therefore, take up the full armor of God, so that you will be able to resist in the evil day, and having done everything, to stand firm." Ephesians 6:12, 13

This chapter will deal with breaking a spiritual attack that is associated with most, if not all, cancers. We see a number of times in the Bible where afflictions in the body are associated with attacks by spiritual forces of wickedness as described in the above Scripture.

The following Scripture speaks about an enemy: "Be of sober {spirit,} be on the alert. Your adversary, the devil, prowls around like a roaring lion, seeking someone to devour." 1 Peter 5:8

Jesus Himself said, "The thief comes only to steal and kill and destroy; I came that they may have life, and have {it} abundantly." John 10:10

Also He said, "Behold, I have given you authority to tread on serpents and scorpions, and over all the power of the enemy, and nothing will injure you.

Nevertheless do not rejoice in this, that the spirits are subject to you, but rejoice that your names are recorded in heaven." Luke 10:19,20

Chapter 5   Breaking the power of the spirit of Cancer

Although there is an enemy, Jesus came to set us free from his attacks! Praise God !!!

Acts 10: 38 reveals this with these words, "You know of Jesus of Nazareth, how God anointed Him with the Holy Spirit and with power, and how He went about doing good and healing all who were oppressed by the devil, for God was with Him."

We see an example in Scripture of one such affliction caused by an spiritual attack in the following verses:

"And there was a woman who for eighteen years had had a sickness caused by a spirit; and she was bent double, and could not straighten up at all. When Jesus saw her, He called her over and said to her, 'Woman, you are freed from your sickness.' And He laid His hands on her; and immediately she was made erect again and {began} glorifying God." Luke 13:11-13

"And this woman, a daughter of Abraham as she is, whom satan has bound for eighteen long years, should she not have been released from this bond on the Sabbath day?" Luke 13:16

These spiritual attacks were taken care of by Jesus on the cross and today we too are able to be released from any bondages and afflictions Satan may try to attack us with also.

Chapter 5   Breaking the power of the spirit of Cancer

An understanding of a spiritual attack associated with cancer came to me by way of the Holy Spirit speaking as I continued to seek Him for more understanding.

I heard the Holy Spirit speak to me and say, **"The life is in the blood"!**
I began asking Him over and over for a period of time what this had to do with cancer.

As I sought Him, He quickened the Scripture to me, " the thief (Satan) comes only to steal, and kill and destroy; I came that they might have life, and might have it abundantly." John 10:10

He then revealed that in cancer there is an attack of the enemy to **"steal the blood".**

He used an example of something that happened to me to explain this to me.

While praying for people with cancer in our ministry the "Divine Healing Rooms- Seattle Eastside"; I developed some warts on my left hand. I had the thought I needed to get those burnt off or something. Then the Holy Spirit convicted me of believing for people to be healed of cancer and yet I wasn't even going to pray against these three little warts, a small form of cancer in themselves.

So, I cursed the three warts in Jesus Name and commanded them to die and fall off. In about three weeks they all dried up and fell off and have not come back in over a year.
Praise God! I was rejoicing and hoping to see full-fledged cancers do the same!

Chapter 5   Breaking the power of the spirit of Cancer

Later on, another wart appeared on my right hand. So, I prayed the same way against it as I had done with the other three warts but nothing happened. I kept praying but nothing changed. So, I began seeking God as to why this one didn't die and fall off like the other ones.

One day at one of my son's baseball games the wart was irritating me and seemed to have developed a piece of it in the center that stuck up more. As the game went on it seemed to itch and was just begging for me to yank it out. So, finally I pinched that part in the middle and pulled it out. Once out it looked like a "plug". As soon as I pulled it out blood began to pour out. I thought 'what have I done now'? I felt pretty silly but stopped the blood and as I was looking at the mess the Holy Spirit began to speak to me.

He said, **"the life is in the blood, without blood and its nourishing nutrients the cancer can't live and grow; it steals the blood, if you pull the plug on the blood, the cancer can't live and will die."**

Then a few days later another incident happened. I was downstairs in our basement checking on some water that was leaking in from some heavy rains. There is a drain in the floor to remove any water that might leak in. As I was checking on it I noticed that it was positioned in such a way that the water was not draining from it. When I lifted up the cover the water all rushed down the drain. The Holy Spirit reminded me of the center plug in the wart and how when I pulled it the blood all flowed out. He said, **"You have to pull the plug on cancer, remove the plug and it will drain away like the water."**

Chapter 5   Breaking the power of the spirit of Cancer

Time went on and I began to notice the wart that was on my right hand, without me doing anything to it, was beginning to shrink and diminish. As more time went on it completely fell apart, broke off bit-by-bit and disappeared and has not returned.

Again, I heard the Holy Spirit speak to me, "the life is in the blood". I continued seeking to understand. What was the plug of cancer? What did that centerpiece of my wart represent in cancer? The removing of the drain cover, what does that represent?

It was truly amazing how by that "plug" being removed the wart just died seemingly by itself with no other action on my part.

I continued just seeking the Lord about these things trying to grasp and understand about this "stealing of the blood" by cancer and "how to pull the plug" on the blood supply to the cancer. As time went on and no more came I prayed only what I knew up to that point in the Divine Healing Rooms for people with cancer. I trusted that as I moved in what God had given that He would be faithful to give more.

As we prayed for people with cancer among other things I would pray, " In the Name of Jesus I come against every operation and attack of Satan to steal the blood for the cancer cells and I bind up these attacks and cut off the blood to the cancer cells in the Name of Jesus."

Chapter 5   Breaking the power of the spirit of Cancer

As time went on in ministry I began doing more praying for people with cancer and we opened up a new ministry called the "Cancer Healing Rooms" to develop the fight against cancer.

One part of that ministry was to hold "Cancer Seminars" where we would teach and minister the things the Lord had shown us and also pray for healing for those fighting cancer.

The first "Cancer Seminar" was scheduled for May 18, 2004 on a Tuesday. Our plan was to use all that the Lord had given us up to that point to minister to the people coming and trust God to give more as we were obedient to steward what we had.

The night before the first Cancer Seminar, Monday night, May 17, 2004, just as I laid down to go to sleep, I found myself in a very real dream. Normally I don't dream much or I don't remember them if I do, but this one I did.

This was the dream that I still remember very vividly: I was sitting in a large room, like a church auditorium, in the front row talking with some other people. Someone then walked up to me and asked if I would go up to the front platform area and pray for a boy who had cancer.

I said "yes" and walked up to the boy. Some others were standing around also. The boy appeared to be maybe 11 or 12 years old and looked normal. I began to pray against the cancer and suddenly out from his feet an ugly looking creature lurched out and began circling around and around me and the boy.

Chapter 5   Breaking the power of the spirit of Cancer

I found myself no longer dealing with the boy but with this ugly, ugly distorted terrible looking creature that was slithering and wiggling around me. It moved like a snake and was covered in a slimy material like a newt. It had the general appearance of a crocodile or alligator in size and shape and was covered in strong pointed spikes like big crocodiles usually have.

It was different in that instead of a mouth in front, like crocodiles have, the mouth was on top of its head and it looked like a blood sucking leech's mouth with lots of teeth all wiggling and looking for something to latch onto.

I found myself in a spiritual battle with this thing trying to get it to go and disappear! It was like a wrestling match; it did not want to go. I used all the Scriptures I knew and every spiritual warfare tool I knew. I was getting tired and it was still just wiggling around my feet. It never seemed to try to attack me or the boy it just wiggled around us on and on.

Finally in the dream I saw myself shout, " Satan, in Jesus Name I rebuke you- Go!" It went; it disappeared in front of my eyes. I immediately woke up from the dream.

Chapter 5   Breaking the power of the spirit of Cancer

I don't know what the boy in the dream did or anything else because it was over and I was sitting up in bed tired and a little worn out from the battle. I went in the living room and got something to eat to refresh myself and relax a little and began to ponder the dream.

This appeared to be a demonic spirit that came out of the boy with cancer.

I believed the timing of it coincided with the Cancer Seminar being the next morning and that God was giving me more insight into things. Since it appeared to be half leech or lamprey and half crocodile I decided to look up leech on the Internet to see what I could find.

The blood sucking attaching mouth on the top of its head was definitely its outstanding unusual feature besides just being awful to look at and watch. It was interesting to read the definition of a leech on the Internet: "Any of various chiefly aquatic bloodsucking annelid worms once used by physicians to bleed their patients; (2) one who preys on or lives off others, clings to another, parasite, to drain the essence or exhaust the resources of its host."

This dream, I believe, was from God to show me that there is also a spiritual attack involved in cancer that must be broken.

The dream seemed to reveal that the demonic creature I saw come out of the boy was linked to his cancer. The blood sucking mouth seemed to reveal that this creature was used to somehow "steal the blood" from the boy and use it for its own purposes- for the cancer cells to have the "life of the blood" and to grow off its host.

Chapter 5   Breaking the power of the spirit of Cancer

Also the dream revealed that this was a very well protected, strong, armored, and formidable enemy that did not leave easily, thus bringing a partial understanding of why cancer has been so difficult to see healed in the past.

The next day in the Cancer Seminar, as well as covering everything else, we came against this spiritual attack for those attending the seminar.

Another piece of the puzzle had been revealed. Through the Holy Spirit speaking about the "life is in the blood" and the wart and drain illustrations I knew He had revealed what this thing was that was involved in the <u>stealing of the blood for the cancer</u>- the demonic spirit with an appearance of a crocodile and a leech that came out of the boy.

It seemed to make sense that to remove this demonic spirit would be likened to pulling out the centerpiece in my wart or the drain cover in the basement. It made sense that if that demonic spirit were removed that the blood supply to the cancer cells would dry up and hopefully the cancer would dry up and die and fall off just like my wart did.

So, I began to pray this way for those fighting cancer. I rebuked this thing stealing the blood and commanded it to go. I didn't know what to call it, a spirit of pride, a spirit of cancer, a spirit of death, a thief, who knows?; so I called it all of those things and started commanding it to leave in Jesus Name.

Chapter 5   Breaking the power of the spirit of Cancer

I continued seeking the Lord about this dream and the demonic creature and how it was used to steal the blood. Also, I sought the Lord as to what gave it the right to attack, and in the dream, to enter into the boy with cancer.

Thank God for all the intercessors and folks praying for God to give more understanding to us about all these things. They are the faithful ones behind the scenes causing God's mercy and grace to be released to the church.

Another piece of the puzzle, more understanding, was to come on June 7, 2004.

I was praying for the Cancer Seminar students in my office that day and coming against that spirit of cancer, or pride, or whatever it was, and rebuking it in Jesus Name.

As I was rebuking it, I found coming up from my heart and then out of my mouth the word - "Leviathan" . I continued praying and rebuking "Leviathan". I didn't know why that word suddenly popped out of my mouth like that while I was praying. I had not been reading or studying anything about that name or ever had that I could remember.

I put it on the back shelf and finished my prayer time. It was a busy day and I just continued on not thinking anything more about it as it didn't really mean anything to me.

Chapter 5   Breaking the power of the spirit of Cancer

Later that night while sitting in the living room with my wife studying for the Tuesday Evening Divine Healing Rooms meeting, I remembered what had happened. I mentioned it to Joy, my wife, and we talked about it and wondered what it meant. As we talked, we decided to look it up in Scripture and see if the Lord might speak to us.

We remembered it being in Job somewhere so we looked it up. We found the word "Leviathan" in Job chapter 41. The whole chapter was about Leviathan. As I started to read it we prayed and asked the Holy Spirit to speak to us through the verses if there was something He was trying to speak to us through this word.

We did not have to read far! Job 41:1 says, "Can you draw out Leviathan with a fishhook?"
There was a side margin note on the word "Leviathan" so I glanced over to see what they had to say about the word. It read: "Or, the crocodile" That got our attention! The dream of the boy with cancer came back very vividly at the moment! Wow! Leviathan, the crocodile! Our minds started racing! It seemed God was revealing more.

We read on and were amazed as all the verses in Job chapter 41 began describing this creature and its characteristics. It reminded me over and over of things in the dream as to this creature's nature. I stopped and said to my wife, let's believe God as we read on that if this is indeed the biblical, spiritual name of that demonic creature I saw in the dream that something will dramatically confirm it by what we read.

Chapter 5   Breaking the power of the spirit of Cancer

As we read on nothing seemed to click in a dramatic way. Then at the very end, in the last verse in the chapter were awesome words that confirmed to us that this word "Leviathan" was the name of the crocodile, leech type spirit associated with the boy and with cancer.

Job 41: 34: "He looks on everything that is high; He is King over all the sons of pride."

"King over the sons of pride" – Wow! I couldn't believe my eyes! There it is!
The word "pride" - the spiritual root sin of cancer in the same chapter speaking of Leviathan and his nature; but there was much more.

Leviathan "looks on everything that is high" – what does that mean? It speaks of him looking around, scouting around, searching for and attracted to everything and anyone that is "high". What is "high"? It speaks of pride! Like someone who goes around with their nose stuck up in the air all the time! In Isaiah 14: 13,14 we read of Satan saying, " I will ascend to heaven; I will raise my throne above the stars of God, …I will ascend above the heights of the clouds; I will make myself like the Most High."

"Leviathan" is looking on everything that is high because he is attracted to pride!

Chapter 5　　　　　Breaking the power of the spirit of Cancer

Pride catches his eyes and he goes to and is attracted to it because that pride is what opens the door for him to be able to come in and attack his prey. He is like the one Peter spoke of when he said, "Be on the alert, Your adversary, the devil, prowls about like a roaring lion, seeking someone to devour." 1 Peter 5: 8

"Leviathan" needs a door opened to be able to attack his prey. Something gives him the legal right to be able to come in and steal, kill and destroy. Jesus said of Satan that he came but not finding anything in Jesus left for a more opportune time! Luke 4:13 says, "When the devil had finished every temptation, he left Him until an opportune time."

Where Satan finds the generational sin of pride passed down through the forefathers and in an individual person, he is allowed to attack. Not only does he attack but God's Word says that "He is King over all the sons of pride". He becomes 'King' over them!

He begins to rule and control!

"Leviathan" comes in and affects the physical body. We see an example of this being possible through Jesus' ministry. Luke 13:11,13 says, "And there was a woman who for eighteen years had had a sickness caused by a spirit; and she was bent double, and could not straighten up at all… And He laid His hands on her; and immediately she was made erect again and {began} glorifying God."

Chapter 5   Breaking the power of the spirit of Cancer

"Leviathan" doesn't cause someone to be physically bent over, this spirit comes to "steal the blood" from its host like a parasite and reroute it to already lawless cancerous cells to cause them to multiply even faster with an abundant supply of blood.

Only later on after praying against this operation to "steal the blood" because "the life is in the blood" did I discover from a cancer patient in the Divine Healing Rooms one night that he was on a new treatment that seeks to cut off the blood supply to the tumors. He also shared something else I did not know then, that cancer as it grows develops and forms its own ever-larger blood vessels to get more blood to feed on. That right there confirms that there is something beyond the natural order dictating and controlling and directing this stealing of the blood!

Now I understand more than ever why it has been so hard to set people free from cancer.
When you read all of chapter 41 in Job, you read a description of a creature that is a very formidable foe. It is described in length with many details to bring across its mighty defenses and power.

(See Appendix F to read the Scriptures relating to Leviathan in Job 41.)

Now we know the enemy- that is most of the battle! The good news is that Jesus came to set us free from all the attacks of Satan and his household.

Chapter 5   Breaking the power of the spirit of Cancer

Jesus said some very, very encouraging words to us;

"The seventy returned with joy, saying, 'Lord, even the demons are subject to us in Your name.' And He said to them, 'I was watching Satan fall from heaven like lightning.'

'Behold, I have given you authority to tread on serpents and scorpions, and over all the power of the enemy, and nothing will injure you.
     Nevertheless do not rejoice in this, that the spirits are subject to you, but rejoice that your names are recorded in heaven.'

At that very time He rejoiced greatly in the Holy Spirit, and said, 'I praise You, O Father, Lord of heaven and earth, that You have hidden these things from {the} wise and intelligent and have revealed them to infants. Yes, Father, for thus it was well-pleasing in Your sight." Luke 10:17-21

Jesus came and gave us, as believers, the power and authority over demon spirits. You as a believer in Jesus, using your God given authority, can rebuke in Jesus name "Leviathan" and command that spirit of cancer to go from you!

Jesus said in Mark 16,17: "These signs will accompany those who have believed: in My name they will cast out demons..." As you repent of the sin of pride and submit to God and His will and receive forgiveness of your sin, you gain the authority and power to rebuke this spirit of cancer, this Leviathan from stealing your blood anymore and can command it to go from you.

Chapter 5   Breaking the power of the spirit of Cancer

Another "piece of the puzzle" came as the Holy Spirit began to impress me with the need to "bind the strong man." I was familiar with this term. It refers to Jesus' words in the gospels of the need to "bind the strong man" in certain cases to set people free of spiritual demonic attacks.

I began to seek the Lord as to what the "strong man" of cancer was that we needed to bind.

As I sought the Lord about this, after some time, I heard the Holy Spirit speak to me and say "the strong man of death." This made sense to me right away. Death is the overall outcome Satan seeks to bring about by the spiritual attacks of Leviathan and others. The strong man tries to bring about the "fear of death" from the cancer and ultimately death itself. While all this was going on, I looked up and began to study more the words of Jesus about first "binding the strong man."

Jesus spoke about this need to first "bind the strong man" up in Mark 3: 27 and Luke 11:21, 22. This "strong man of death" must first of all be bound up in order to remove the attacking demonic "spirit of cancer" known as "Leviathan", or fear, infirmity and anything else trying to attack you.

The "strong man" works along the same lines as its name. It is the strong one, the holding force, and the controlling force behind the other demonic spirits. He empowers them to be able to maintain their position in our body to carry on their work. When the "strong man" is bound, the other "lesser spirits" lose strength and "staying power" and can be removed from the person or "house" as referred to by Jesus.

Chapter 5   Breaking the power of the spirit of Cancer

Jesus said in Mark 3: 27, "But no one can enter the strong man's house (our body's) and plunder (remove) his property (lesser demons the strong man controls) unless he first binds the strong man, and then he will plunder his house."

This same teaching by Jesus is seen also in Luke 11: 17-26. "But if I cast out demons by the finger of God, then the kingdom of God has come upon you. When a strong man, fully armed, guards his own house, his possessions are undisturbed. But when someone stronger than he attacks him and overpowers him, he takes away from him all his armor on which he had relied and distributes his plunder."

God's Word tells us, "You are from God, little children, and have overcome them; because greater is He who is in you than he who is in the world (satan and his demons)." 1 John 4:4 The Holy Spirit in you is greater than any strong man attacking you or any spirit of cancer and able to bind them up and remove them from attacking you any longer.

Thus, taking our rightful authority given to us by God's Word we need to "bind the strong man" of death and strip him of his protective armor so that he can be removed along with his lesser attacking spirits of cancer, Leviathan, fear, etc. What is the strong man's armor that we need to "take away" as Jesus said. The armor is "sin". What sin? Again, the "sin of pride", lawlessness, "taking on a life of our own", and seeking to live our own will, not seeking after God's will for our life.

Chapter 5   Breaking the power of the spirit of Cancer

We remove his armor and bind him up and gain the ability to remove the spirit of cancer-Leviathan, etc. by repenting, (turning away, not doing it anymore) confessing our sin of pride, and asking God to forgive us and to wash us in the blood of Jesus.

This removes his legal right to attack us. Gods' Word says, "And they overcame him because of the blood of the Lamb and because of the word of their testimony,…" Revelation 12:11

As you receive the blood of Jesus for the forgiveness of your sins and the word of your testimony is that you have repented and turned away from the sin of pride, the sin of " taking on a life of your own", of living for your "own will", not God's will, you become the "overcomer" of the "strong man" and strip him of his "armor" and "bind" him up and are able to command him to go from you and along with his "property" (the spirit of Leviathan, cancer, fear, infirmity etc.)

After removing the strong mans' armor through prayer and taking our authority to bind up the "strong man of death" by the Name of Jesus, we are ready to "plunder" or "take out" the lesser demonic spirits attacking us. We now command in the Name of Jesus that the spirit of cancer, Leviathan, fear, infirmity, and anything else you are aware of to "go", "leave", and be removed from you and not return.

We take our stand on Jesus' words, "Behold, I have given you authority to tread on serpents and scorpions, and over all the power of the enemy, and nothing will injure you." Luke 10:19

Chapter 5   Breaking the power of the spirit of Cancer

You must fight, take a stand on God's Word, fight for your life, your loved ones, be strong, rise up, be bold, be an overcomer as Jesus called you to be.

Take your God given authority, put God's Words in your mouth, use the Name of Jesus with power and authority, be a fighter, take command and take this knowledge given to you and fight using the blood of Jesus and the "Name of Jesus" to rebuke these attacks on your life.

Jesus gave "you" authority to tread on, to destroy these scorpions and serpents (cancer) so rise up and do it. Don't be concerned about saying or doing this "spiritual warfare" the right way, there is no formula, just rise up, let a "holy" anger come up in you and begin to pray and speak forth, the Holy Spirit will come alongside and help you fight and overcome.

There is a prayer for this spiritual warfare in the next chapter, use this as a guideline, but go beyond it as the Lord leads you, let as much spiritual, Holy Spirit power and "force" as you can rise up in you.

You can do it! God will help you! Go ahead take your place of authority! Be bold! Be strong!

In repentance and forgiveness you also gain the authority to speak to those cancer cells and command them to die and leave your body and speak to every cell in your body to STOP "taking on a life of its own" and come back into divine order.

Chapter 5   <u>Breaking the power of the spirit of Cancer</u>

You can receive healing in your body from Jesus from all the damage the cancer may have done and be made whole by Jesus.

Although God's anointing and the gift of healing can operate to totally deliver you from cancer in a moments time, most healing takes place as we believe and act on God's Word.

You don't have to go to a miracle crusade although they are fine and we encourage you to go if the Lord leads you.

You also can pray yourself, or better, ask a group of believers to stand in agreement with you and pray for healing and deliverance from cancer with this knowledge.

The Holy Spirit may also give you more insights and particular aspects for you in breaking the power of cancer over your life.

Chapter 6

Prayer for Healing of Cancer - Part 2

Prayer for healing and deliverance from Cancer!

Heavenly Father, I come to you in the Name of Jesus! I come crying out for mercy and grace in time of need. Have mercy on me, forgive me of my sins! I need you and I invite you into my life.

Forgive me of the sin of pride. I repent and I turn to follow you, to seek after Your Will in my life each and every day. I ask you to forgive my forefathers, my ancestors, of the sin of pride. I remit to you all the sins of previous generations in my family and ask you to forgive them and wash away our sins in the blood of Jesus.

I renounce all self-determination pride, lawlessness, selfish ambition, being controlling, and controlling the outcomes of people and situations and will seek you constantly for Your will in my life and I submit myself to you now and forever.

I turn to say like Jesus, "not my will but Your will be done".

I ask you to wash me in the Blood of Jesus and cleanse me from all sin. I receive the shed blood of Jesus and His sacrifice for my sins and sicknesses.

Chapter 6   Prayer for Healing of Cancer – Part 2

Thank you Jesus for taking my sins on the cross and my sicknesses, I come to you as my Savior as my Deliverer and I ask you to heal me and set me free from all cancer.

I receive healing in my body now and thank you for healing me.

Now in the Name of Jesus, I speak to every lawless, rebellious cancerous cell in my body and I command you to die and leave my body in Jesus Name. I rebuke you in Jesus Name and command you to stop taking on a life of your own and to come back into divine order.

You have lost your legal right to take on a life of your own as I am no longer taking on a life of my own and in Jesus Name I command you to stop, die, leave, go, be removed from my body. I rebuke cancer, sickness, death, and every attack of cancer in Jesus Name.

I receive the life of Jesus, the abundant life of the Lord Jesus in me right now. "By His stripes I was healed" and I receive my blood bought healing now in Jesus Name.

Now in Jesus Name, I bind up the "strong man of death" as Jesus said and I plunder your household. I rebuke the spirit of cancer,

Leviathan, the spirit of infirmity, the spirit of death and every foul demonic spirit attacking me and command it to go in Jesus Name. It is written, in My Name you will cast out demons and I cast you out now Satan and all your household in Jesus Name.

Chapter 6   Prayer for Healing of Cancer – Part 2

Go Satan, and do not return! "Get the behind me Satan"! "The Lord rebuke you Satan"! I plead the blood of Jesus between you and me and give you no place! It is written, "the destroyer will not pass through the blood" and I receive the blood of Jesus over me, on me, and around me now.

Heavenly Father, fill me now with your Holy Spirit, come and fill me up with You! I receive your love, joy, and peace.

I receive and embrace humility in my life. I ask you to help me walk humbly before you and I thank you now for healing me and setting me free.

Come, speak to me and show me Your plan, Your will, Your destiny for my life. I turn to follow you just as Jesus said.

Show me where you are going and what you are doing so that I can be with you where you are.

Make my life what it ought to be.

Thank you Father in Jesus Name! Amen, Amen and Amen!

Chapter 7

Walking in Humility and God's Will

God's Word!

"After He had removed him, He raised up David to be their king, concerning whom He also testified and said, 'I HAVE FOUND DAVID the son of Jesse, a man After My Heart, who will do all My will."
Acts 13:22

Prayer Time!
Heavenly Father, I ask you to change my heart. Put a right heart in me, a heart of humility, a heart that loves you, a heart that seeks after you.

Thank you Father in Jesus Name.

Proclaim Over and Over out Loud!

" He sent His word and healed them, and delivered {them} from their destructions."
Psalm 107:20

Chapter 7   Walking in humility and God's Will

Humility is the antidote for pride! I want to encourage you in your healing to embrace humility as a protection against pride. Leviathan does not look upon humility, nor become King over the sons of humility. He looks the other way for someone else!

"God is opposed to the proud, but gives grace to the humble." James 4:6

God loves you !!! He wants to give us the abundant life Jesus paid the price for.

He doesn't want to see His children suffer the consequences of sin.

Jesus said, "Behold, you have become well; do not sin anymore, so that nothing worse happens to you." John 5:14

As you receive healing and walk in your healing and embrace the seeking of God's will in your life, you will protect yourself against the sin of pride so that it will not come back, and as Jesus said, nothing worse would happen to you.

Jesus also sought to deliver us from the sin of pride and its consequences when he said these words, "For whoever wishes to save his life will lose it, but whoever loses his life for My sake and the gospel's will save it." Mark 8:35

It's in laying down our will, our own life and seeking the life God has for us that we receive the greatest joy and ultimate rewards.

Chapter 7   Walking in humility and God's Will

We need to take seriously this issue of yielding to God's will and not "barreling ahead in life" as if God did not have a will for our life. We see below in these words of Jesus that we can know the Lord and yet not do His will and face the penalty. In order to "do His will" we must actively seek His will and find out what it is.

Too many of us run through life with scarcely a moment of time left over to seek the Lord for His will and purposes for us. Sometimes we are just too busy doing our will, living as if there is no God! It's not too late to change!

Jesus warns us, "Not everyone who says to Me, 'Lord, Lord,' will enter the kingdom of heaven, but he who does the will of My Father who is in heaven {will enter.}" Matthew 7:21

God will reveal His will to us as we seek Him diligently and enable us to be able to do His will in our life!

We need to be more like Jesus, speaking of Him the Scriptures say, " THEN I SAID, 'BEHOLD, I HAVE COME (IN THE SCROLL OF THE BOOK IT IS WRITTEN OF ME) TO DO YOUR WILL, O GOD." Hebrews 10:7

He has a promise also for us as we seek and yield to His Will; "For you have need of endurance, so that when you have done the will of God, you may receive what was promised." Hebrews 10:36

Chapter 7   Walking in humility and God's Will

There is a powerful promise of God found in 1 Peter 5:5-7, "and all of you, clothe yourselves with humility toward one another, for GOD IS OPPOSED TO THE PROUD, BUT GIVES GRACE TO THE HUMBLE.

Therefore humble yourselves under the mighty hand of God, that He may exalt you at the proper time, casting all your anxiety on Him, because He cares for you."

It's a good place to be "under" God, to be submitted to Him constantly instead of "high" and an open target for the enemy. God gives grace to us when we are not proud. Grace is like the oil in a car engine; it's hard to run an engine without oil, you won't go very far.

Humility is submitting to God, being obedient to Him from the heart, living a life dependent upon Him and not acting independently as if there were no God to live for.

Humility thinks and cares about others needs and situations. Pride is self-centered and self is always the subject of the conversation. Humility looks to do things as a team; it seeks unity and group input and feedback. Pride seeks to function alone, to act independently without consulting others and seeks to isolate itself and act alone. Humility is warm, open, and open hearted to others. Pride is offish, cool to others, and ignores others.

Humility encourages others, reaches out to others interests, and asks questions about others.

Pride always turns the conversation back to self, self-activities, self-projects, and self-accomplishments.

Chapter 7   Walking in humility and God's Will

Humility is honest, forthright, transparent and secure. Pride is deceitful, always seeking to keep things hidden, under cover, protected from accountability, and a "nobody's going to tell me" attitude.

Humility confesses easily any mistakes or errors. Pride covers up, makes excuses, and seeks to always justify any mistakes. Humility rejoices in others accomplishments and successes. Pride envies others being promoted or recognized. Humility wants to learn, is teachable, and looks to others for insights and wisdom. Pride knows it all, only wants to tell others how it will be done, and makes declarations and controlling statements all the time.

Humility seeks to serve and bless others, give acknowledgements to others, and gives encouragement to others. Pride is self-absorbed, seeks to be served, be waited on, and receive praise. Humility submits to others and authority. Pride resists authority through others. Humility asks for correction and help. Pride fights correction and never wants others to see any weakness or failures.

Humility is happy to be unknown, unseen, in the background, and hidden. Pride seeks to be seen, be recognized, be honored, and be acknowledged, to sit in the front, to be the first.

Just as "high" and "pride" attracts Satan to attack and afflict us, the opposite, humility attracts God to us and He promises to bless us with Grace, exalt us in proper time and many other promises.

God is looking too! He is looking on everyone embracing humility to come and be your King;
a King that blesses you with abundant life! God is good! Glory to His Name! Amen!

Chapter 8

Healing of the heart from Pride

God's Word!

"Behold, I will bring to it health and healing, and I will heal them;
and I will reveal to them an abundance of peace and truth." Jeremiah 33: 6

Prayer Time!

Heavenly Father, I ask you to heal my heart. I ask you to place the Father's Heart of Love in my heart, to remove all abandonment, any orphan spirit remaining in me and restore to me that sense of being secure
in My Father's Love.

Thank you Father in Jesus Name.

Proclaim Over and Over out Loud!

"Heal me, O Lord, and I will be healed."
Jeremiah 17: 14

The Father's Love for us not only wants to heal us from the cancer but Father God wants to heal our hearts of anything rooted deep down in it that would open the door for pride and self-determination to enter in.

In the process of bringing us into repentance, healing and making us whole, God wants to not only forgive any sin in our life but to set us free from any and all influence's that may have opened the door to sin. Sometimes there are generational sins pressuring us to fall into a sin over and over again.

Jesus comes to set us free as we cry out to Him to deliver us.

Sometimes there are hurts, offenses, and experiences that open a door for a weakness to enter in. These can cause a corresponding reaction of pride, self-will, and lawlessness.

These experiences are common to all and there is no condemnation in Christ Jesus if you have experienced some of these in your life; yet God wants to heal you!

One area in particular that seems to bring about the sin of pride, self-will, and self- determination is a lack of the sense of the Father's Love in a person's life.

When someone has not received the Father's Heart and Love, there is a sense of abandonment, of being an orphan, and the tendency to act independently, even rebelliously and lawlessly.

Chapter 8 _____ Healing of the heart from Pride

Jesus spoke of this when He said,

"I will not leave you as orphans; I will come to you." John 14:18
Jesus continued in verse 20 to reveal His answer to that orphan
tendency, He said, " In that day you shall know that I am in My
Father, and you in Me, and I in you."

There is a sense of security when God is close; in fact His
plan was to be "in you" to remove any sense of abandonment or
orphan feeling.

Let's come to God now and ask Him to heal us of any weak
spots in our soul or hurts from the past or any other thing that
might have caused us to turn towards living a self-willed, lawless
way of life.

Cancer Healing Prayer – Father's Love

Heavenly Father, I come to you in Jesus Name. I ask you to
heal me. I call upon your Name and ask for your mercy and grace
to come to me now and set me free from anything in my heart or
life that is a root cause of self-will pride in my life.

I ask you to forgive me of any sin, any rebellion in my heart,
of living a self-willed life. Forgive me, my family, my parents, and
their parents, going back three to four generations of the sin of
self-will pride. Set me free, deliver me, and heal my heart and soul.

I renounce all self-will, pride, self-determination, and
lawlessness in my life and repent of it and turn from it now. I
invite you Jesus into everything I ever experienced in my life and
ask you to come into it and set me free and heal me.

Chapter 8   Healing of the heart from Pride

I ask you Father to wash me in the blood of Jesus, wash me with the water of your Word and change, regenerate me, renew me and create in me a clean heart; "sustain me with a willing spirit."
(Psalm 51:12)

I ask you Father to fill me with the Father's Love, give me your Father's Heart, and remove far from me any sense of being abandoned or being an orphan. I receive your love and ask according to your Word, " that I may be filled up to all the fullness of God." (Ephesians 3:19)

I ask you also according to your Word that, " I may be filled with the knowledge of His will in all spiritual wisdom and understanding, so that I may walk in a manner worthy of the Lord, to please Him in all respects, bearing fruit in every good work and increasing in the knowledge of God;" (Colossians 1:9-10)

Father God, I trust you to speak to me, to reveal to me Your will as I seek you diligently that I may walk in humility and fulfill your plan and destiny for my life. I am your servant and will daily come before you and ask you to reveal Your will, Your life to me that I may walk humbly before you all the days of my life and one day hear you say those words to me, "Well done, good and faithful slave;... enter into the joy of your master." (Matthew 25:23)

"Blessed is the man who listens to Me, watching daily at my gates, waiting at my doorsteps. For he who finds Me finds life, and obtains favor from the Lord. But he who sins against me injures himself;..." (Proverbs 8:34-36)

Chapter 8   Healing of the heart from Pride

Healing many times is a process so do not be discouraged if you experience the Holy Spirit healing you and rooting out weaknesses over a period of time.

Finish the race, do not quit or be discouraged. Keep holding fast to the promises of God. Keep looking to Jesus the Author and Finisher of your faith. (Hebrews 12:2) "Suddenly's" happen in the kingdom of God.

At the darkest hour many times light breaks forth.

God is good; His mercy is new every day.

He loves you so don't give up because of what you hear, see or feel; keep your eyes and heart on God's Word until what you hear, see and feel changes to be what God's Word says.

"The Lord bless you and keep you and make His face shine on you and be gracious to you and give you peace."

(Numbers 6:24-26)

Chapter 9

Prayers for Healing & Repentance

Jesus, "Son of David, Have mercy on me!"
Have mercy, Have mercy! Have mercy on me!

Heavenly Father, I come to you now in the name of Jesus.

I ask you to reveal yourself to me;

I invite you to come into my life, my heart, my soul, and my body.

I give you permission to minister to me; I open my heart to you
and cry out for your   mercy and grace to come to me now,
I ask You to speak to me   (Matthew 4:4).

I need you, I ask you Holy Spirit to come to me now to reveal your
love, your Presence and your healing power in my life.

You said in Your Word that "mercy triumphs over judgment";
(James 2:13)
So Heavenly Father I ask You for Your Mercy to come now and
reveal and remove any and all judgments in my life that may be
enabling cancer in my body or keeping You from granting me
repentance and forgiveness of any sin or judgments that may be
hindering my healing and deliverance.

Chapter 9   Prayers for Healing & Repentance

Heavenly Father, I cry out - "deliver me from evil !"

I humbly come before you acknowledging that I have fallen short of your perfect will for my life and I ask you now to forgive me of my sins and my past family line of their sins and to set me free from any effects of sin in my life.

I ask you to forgive me now of any lawlessness in my life, any self-willed life style, any self-centered ambitious lifestyle, any self-ambition pride.

Forgive me now of in any way trying to be God by controlling circumstances, controlling the outcome of events, controlling events in my life and other people's lives, or trying to control the future.

Forgive me for saying things like "I'll never this or that" or "I will be this or that" or "that will never happen to me", or "I'll never get cancer" or any other any type of the "I will" type of statements found in James 4:13-16 as if I were God and could control my life or others' lives or the future.

I renounce any self-will pride, selfish ambition and lawlessness and anything and everything that is not pleasing to you God and ask you to reveal any such thing to me and set me free from it.

Chapter 9   Prayers for Healing & Repentance

I ask you Heavenly Father to forgive my past family generations of the sin of pride and self-willed ambition; forgive them Father, they didn't know what they were doing.

I receive the precious blood of Jesus for the forgiveness of my sins and ask you,

Jesus, to wash me with the water of your Word, transforming, renewing and regenerating me.

Heavenly Father, I ask you now in Jesus' Name to come and touch me, heal me, deliver me from this cancer, set me free from all sickness and affliction.

I receive your mercy, your love, your forgiveness and your power and your healing in my body now as a gift from you because Jesus already paid for my healing on the cross.

Thank you Father in Jesus Name!

Declare the words of the section below strongly, with boldness and force and authority!

In the name of Jesus, I break all the power of Satan to come and steal, kill, and destroy my life and command Satan and all his attacks to go from me now!

Chapter 9   Prayers for Healing & Repentance

In the name of Jesus Christ I bind up the strongman of death, and rob his house of every evil thing as Jesus said, I rebuke the spirit of cancer, Leviathan, infirmity, fear and every evil thing and loose it from me and give it no place. I bind up every operation| of the spirit of cancer & Leviathan to steal my blood to feed the cancer and command every blood vessel supplying blood to the cancer cells or tumors to be cut off, shrink, dissolve and removed.

It is written, "Behold I have given you power to tread on serpents and scorpions, and over all the power of the enemy, and nothing shall be any means harm you." (Luke 10:19)

So, in the Name of Jesus Christ of Nazareth, "the Lord rebuke you Satan", "the Lord rebuke you Satan" , "the Lord rebuke you Satan", Go, Go, Go from me now and do not return! (See Jude 1:9) In the Name of Jesus Christ of Nazareth, I loose all the judgments of sin, of the sin of pride and self-will off my life now, being set free from sin and it's judgments by the Blood of Jesus. Yes, Amen !

I rebuke death, I rebuke you cancer, I rebuke you Leviathan (Job 41:34) ,

I rebuke you from harming me, I rebuke you from stealing my blood to feed this cancer and command you to stop, desist now and I command you to go from me, from my body, my life and do not return.

Chapter 9   Prayers for Healing & Repentance

In the name of Jesus, I break every generational curse of pride, selfish ambition, and lawlessness off of me, my family, my children, their children and forever and break the power of any and all ungodly influences being passed down to me and my children.

Jesus, I ask you to come to me now, Lord stretch out your hand to heal me,

I receive your love and healing power flowing into my body now.

Jesus, lead me into your perfect will, your abundant life, I will follow You , Your will be done in my life, not mine anymore!

You be God, You be my Master, My Lord, My King!

I repent from leading a life of my self-will, I ask you to reveal Your Will for my life, Your destiny for me, Your purpose for creating me, Your plans...... " that you may prove what the Will of God is, that which is Good, Acceptable and Perfect." (Romans 12: 2)

Thank you Heavenly Father in Jesus Name' !!! Amen, Amen, and Amen !!!!

Pray this Prayer for Healing from Cancer every day for at least 21 days for a break though !!! (See Daniel 10:13)

Pray this out of your heart and spirit with forcefulness and confidence and eventually let it flow more and more in your own words and heart.

Additional Scriptures to Consider:

Proverbs 3: 7,8: "Fear the Lord and turn away from evil. It will be healing to your body and refreshment to your bones."

See James 3:16 to see why your repentance is a key to your healing - the "disorder" and the "every evil thing" here is the cancer attacking you, all selfish ambition, all self will, all " I " this and " I " that must go!

See Isaiah 14: 13-15 - the allegory of the "5 I will's" that God judges
.

See Jonah 3:10 and Jonah 4:2 to see God's compassion and loving kindness when we repent and like John the Baptist declared, "Bring forth fruit in keeping with repentance. Matthew 3:8

See James 5: 15 & 16 to see the need to confess any sin as it relates to your healing !

   We recommend you to ask someone close to you to lovingly share with you if ever they notice you trying to control the outcome of events, trying to control them or others so that you can immediately turn away from that and give over control to King Jesus, our Lord & Master.

An Important Key to Healing and Word of Encouragement for those Fighting Cancer !

We want to reemphasize the great importance of deep repentance generationally and personally of any self-willed lifestyle, selfish ambition lifestyle, controlling of circumstances, controlling of people, controlling of outcomes of situations versus trusting God to be in charge and control, trying to control the future, trying to control the actions of people, etc.

These are all reflections of lawlessness in the heart, of not letting God be God! God is God, you & I are not !

The opposite of "not my will, but Your Will be done". These are usually very difficult, if not almost impossible for someone to recognize in themselves and they need the loving help of someone close to them to reveal it to them or in their parents or in generations going back.

There are exceptions to this being the cause of the cancer of course and there are causes such as chemical exposures, drugs, etc. but outside of that, we consistently see year after year, person after person, this being a major issue in their lives , and also by those fighting cancer and/or by their spouses, friends, etc.

Chapter 9   Prayers for Healing & Repentance

Where we have seen real sorrow and real deep repentance and the asking of God for forgiveness in these areas for them and their past generations, we have seen the cancer stop in its tracks and retreat, and stay that way.

Also, we have seen many times an initial repentance, etc. for the sake of being healed and living with the wonderful result of the cancer shrinking, be undetectable, stop, etc. and then unfortunately after the good reports and time of being healed the person returning to that self-willed, controlling, selfish ambition lifestyle choices only to see the cancer come back even stronger and faster than before.

So, please pray about and discern in your own situation these things.

A Scripture you can stand on for any radiation, Chemotherapy, or other treatments not to harm you or poison you is: Mark 16:18b: to believe, confess (Romans 10: 8-10) and thank Him for these being blessing and health to your body!

Please send us your Comments and Testimony's from this Book and healing ministry !

Richard & Joy McIlvaine

Email: RichardMcIlvaine@gmail.com

Chapter 10

Seven Keys to Keep Cancer From coming Back

There are 7 Keys I believe the Lord has shown me that if you practice these in your daily life will help prevent cancer from being able to take hold in your body. These are disciplines in the Christian Life that God has already instructed us in the Bible to follow. They were given to me one evening as I sat praying in my room on a Ministry trip to Korea. I had heard the Lord say to me some months before "7 Keys to Preventing Cancer", and had been asking the Lord, what are these keys?

You and I are not just physical matter, we have a body, but it is the "tent" we live in while on this earth. We are first and foremost, a spirit being created by God, and we have a soul, united with our spirit, that lives in this body temporarily. Doctors treat that physical body and fight against Cancer the best they can and have, Praise God, gained great ground in dealing with the physical, chemical, biological aspects of our cells, etc. Yet, our spirit and soul are not separate from our body and affect our body tremendously. Recently medical science has gained more and more understanding of how our soul, which is our mind, will, and emotions, affects our natural body.

It is accepted today that stress, an emotion, part of our soul, worries, and fears, can cause stomach ulcers, physical illness, and disease in our body. This is because our body, spirit and soul are all connected and affect each other. When we hold onto unforgiveness and bitterness in our hearts after time it begins to affect our body. At first it may just cause us to develop a frown all the time, but later on in many cases can cause arthritis in our joints.

The Western, Greek thinking mindset of our culture looks to bring healing by dealing just with the physical, biological, chemical makeup of man. But, we are spirit and soul also, and we have lost our biblical foundation understanding of man that reveals to us that sin also can cause sickness in the body and needs to be dealt with to bring healing to the body.

So many times doctors cut out with surgery the cancer only to have it pop up someplace else later, or come back again. This is because the spiritual root cause of the cancer has not been removed. This book has been written to seek to help you remove any root cause of cancer not only for you but for your children and their children on down the family line.

These 7 Keys are meant to remove any root cause of cancer in our lives. They are disciplines that we grow into as we practice them. They are normal Christianity as it is taught in the Bible, designed by God to bless us in this life and enable us to walk in Divine Health.

They take practice and come bit by bit into our life until they become just normal life to us as God intended. God wants us to adjust ourselves to His instructions, His ways, to bless us abundantly not only in this life but in eternity. Let's yield to Him and let the Holy Spirit transform us into the image of Christ, His goal for us in this life on earth.

(1) Key - The Fear of the Lord

Embracing this Cancer preventer in our life starts by understanding God is God and you and I are not God. This sounds silly of course, we know that, but does our day to day life and decisions reflect that ?   To fear the Lord means to reverence Him, respect Him, honor Him and understand that He is our Creator, that we did not make ourselves and are thus subject to Him, and are not an island unto ourselves, living as if there were no God, making our own life plans without considering He is even there and His plans for us and our destiny. It means knowing our place and not stepping out from being the creation, subject to the One who created us.

" Fear the Lord and turn away from evil, It will be healing to your body, ... Proverbs 3:7 ; Here we see in this Scripture, this instruction for living on planet earth, that what we do in our spirit and soul, our mind, affects our physical body. The lack of the "Fear of the Lord" can make us think we can do what the Lord considers "evil" and get away with it and it not have any consequences in our body, but it doesn't work that way, they are connected.

As we "Fear" (respect, reverence) the Lord, we acknowledge Him as God in our life and consult Him about our life, our decisions, we ask Him for His plans for our life, we ask Him what He created us for on this earth to do to Glorify Him. When we come into "Divine Order" in our heart, we become "lawful" to His instructions and let Him take the lead in our life. As we come into "Divine Order", seeking and doing God's Will, the cells in our body also come into "order" and die when they are supposed to die and thus cancer is prevented.

(2) Key – Humility – Meekness of spirit

Humility is a strong preventer of cancer. Humility is the opposite of pride, the root sin cause of cancer and thus important to practice and develop in our life.

Jesus is a perfect example of humility. In Philippians 2: 3-7, we find insights and real strong keys for preventing cancer in our life. Jesus here is our example for living in Divine Order.

"Do nothing from selfishness or empty conceit, but with humility of mind let each of you regard one another as more important than himself; <u>do not merely look out for your own personal interests, but also for the interests of others.</u> Have this attitude in yourselves which also was in Christ Jesus, who, although He existed in the form of God, did not regard equality with God a thing to be grasped, but <u>EMPTIED HIMSELF</u>, taking the form of a BOND SERVANT, and being made into the likeness of men….He humbled Himself by becoming obedient (to God's Will) to the point of death, even death on a cross."

To come into Divine Order in our lives and in the cells of our body, we too need to become obedient to God, empty ourselves of ourselves and seek to fulfill His plans for us on this earth.

(3) Key – Seeking after God's Will for our life

Another strong medicine to prevent cancer is to constantly be focusing on what is God's Will for me moment by moment in this life. This sets us free from focusing in on the spiritual root cause of cancer – the self-willed, self-determination lifestyle, the sin of pride – self focus instead of being God focused as a way of life.

To give up being self-willed, we need to receive and know God's Will, this comes by seeking Him, and spending time with Him. " The Lord has looked down from Heaven upon the sons of men, to see if there are any who understand , who seek after God, They have all turned aside; together they have become corrupt;...." Psalm 14: 2,3.
We want God to look down from Heaven and see us seeking after Him, and receiving His Will for our lives, knowing His Will will be good, acceptable and perfect as the Scripture says.

" ...that you may prove what the will of God is, that which is good and acceptable, well pleasing and perfect." (Romans 12: 2)

Jesus was our example of living in Divine Order in our lives, what is that order? Jesus said, " Father, if Thou art willing, remove this cup from Me, yet not My Will, but Thine be done." Luke 22:42 God's order is yielding up our will to His, trusting Him as our loving Father that His Will is best and will bless us, be good, and bring us into fulfilling our destiny on this earth and for all of eternity. As we come into Divine Order in our life, divine order will come into our cells and everything else in our life, our marriage's, our children, our finances, our jobs, everything will start to straighten out and flow peacefully with God's Grace and Provision.

(4) Key – Laying down your own life

Practicing on a moment by moment, day by day basis the laying down of your own life for others needs deals a death blow to the self-willed lifestyle root of cancer. This practice keeps us from exerting a self-willed, selfish, self-centered lifestyle. Laying down our life at a moment's notice, giving up our will, and seeking God's Will in every situation delivers us from the spiritual root cause of cancer. Laying down our life means to give up the right to be in control of situations, of the outcome of things, of people in our lives, our money, our time, etc. and instead laying down our life to see what God wants to do in that situation, in that person's life, etc.

Jesus said, "For this reason the Father loves Me, because I lay down My life….."   John 10:17.   As we too lay down our life for God and others as the Holy Spirit leads, the **Father's love and blessings begin to flow abundantly into our lives also**. It's when we "stop", "let go", "give up control", and "our will", that God can then come in and begin to work and bless us body, soul and spirit. We come into Divine Order and so do the cells in our body.

(5) Key –Worshipping God – Ministering and Blessing God for who He is !

Worshipping God and constantly keeping Him as the focus of our heart and mind sets us free from worshipping ourselves by thinking of ourselves all the time. Ministering to Him, singing songs to Him, thanking Him all the time for His blessings, His Gifts, the Good Things He has done for us over and over again sets us free from self-absorption, from centering our life on ourselves.

As we keep in a constant flow of worship and thanksgivings to God, we become more God conscious and can hear better when He speaks and reveals His Will for our life on a moment by moment or daily basis. We begin to say more, "God this" and "God that" instead of "I this" and "I that", delivering us from the pattern of a self-willed lifestyle thus preventing cancer's spiritual root cause in our life.

(6) Key - Serving others !

Serving others - practicing looking at and recognizing the needs of others around us and responding to those needs as the Holy Spirit leads. Entering into a lifestyle of looking around us at other people and situations and noticing what's going on outside of our own interests. Looking to help and serve others as a lifestyle is strong medicine to deliver us from controlling others for our own self-serving interests.

We can develop the practice of looking at other people and thinking, how could I maybe bless them, help them, give them something, how are they doing?, is there anything God that you want to do here for this person? This again delivers us from a lifestyle of thinking people exist to help me get what I need to succeed in life. We want to instead trust God that in serving Him and others that God will bring us into the wonderful life He has for us.

(7) – Key – Led by the Holy Spirit in all we do !

Let Go and Let God lead! Slow down, stop, give up, relax and give the Holy Spirit a chance to speak or impress the Will of God upon our hearts at any given moment. We tend to run around at such a busy pace with our mind full of so many thoughts and things to do that God doesn't have a chance to get a hold of us to reveal His Will, His plans, that which will work good if we listen and let Him lead us. The Holy Spirit has come as our Helper, to reveal the Father's Will, to speak and lead us into the perfect Will of our Father.

"For all who are being led by the Spirit of God, these are the sons of God" .
(Romans 8:14)

As we let go of self-determining our future and what we think is good to do, and stop and listen, the Holy Spirit has a better way, a plan that will work and bring joy and peace and work best. He speaks down in our belly, our spirit, to reveal the Father's Will, to bring order out of chaos, to bring us into Divine Order in all parts of our life – body, soul and spirit. This obedience to let Him be in control, brings obedience also to our cells to be obedient to their God given DNA instructions, thus preventing cancer. (cells out of control, acting on their own, out of order)

Chapter 10

Conclusion – Final Thoughts

God loves you, your family, and your loved ones. He is revealing these things about cancer out of His love and mercy – He cares for you!

Let me share my heart with you.

The suffering I've seen in individuals and families from cancer is heart rending. Because of that, I haven't held anything back in sharing with people seeking healing from cancer or those wanting to prevent cancer.

"Cancer is us", a Seattle newspaper article stated during the time I was seeking God for confirmations on what He had shared about cancer. It is not an outside virus or bacteria or poison that we have ingested that is now afflicting our body. It is us, and because of that, we can do something about it.

The worst thing is not knowing what's wrong, because if we don't know what's wrong, we can't fix it. We can fix cancer because God is revealing what's wrong; that's His part, now it's time for us to do our part with His help and love.

Chapter 11   Conclusion – Final Thoughts

"Cancer is us" – our cells are out of control because we are "out of control." Our part is to no longer be "out of control." We can make a deep, quality decision to no longer be "out of control." God leaves that decision up to us. That is our part. God has given us a "free will."

What do I do? No longer be "out of control," but under the control of God, the way it was meant to be all along from the beginning of creation with Adam and Eve in the Garden of God.

What do I do to prevent cancer? Let God be in control! Let God be God and you NOT! Step down from the throne where you rule, where you are in control and let God have His rightful place where He rules and we follow.

Yes, giving up control of your life and letting God be in control. Truly making Him Savior and Lord, King of Kings, Lord of Lords!

"Shall we not rather be subject to the Father of spirits and live?" (Hebrews 12:9b). Lawlessness, self-determination, and a self-will lifestyle all come out of pride, of lifting ourselves up to be the one in charge of our own life. This really is setting us up to be like God, to be the one in control, in charge. The problem with this is that God is our Creator and thus reserves the right to rule and be in charge and in control of His creation.

Chapter 11   Conclusion – Final Thoughts

He is the One who has said in His Word, the Bible: "Follow Me," (John 21:22) (John 10:27) "...to all those who obey Him (Jesus) the source of Eternal salvation" (Hebrews 5:9), "I have been crucified with Christ and it is no longer I who live but Christ lives in me, and the life I now live I live by faith [listening and believing what God says to me] in the Son of God" (Galatians 2:20), and finally, "Instead you ought to say, 'If the Lord wills, we shall live and also do this and do that'" (James 4:15).

When we disregard God's Word, we enter into "lawlessness," disregarding the instructions of this life and suffer the consequences.

I get frightened for people these days whenever I hear someone say things like, "I'm never going to get cancer," as if we can control the future and have the power to decide that. Really only God can say "never" because He alone retains control of the future and what can and cannot happen.

I get frightened for people when I hear them say things like, "Well, we decided, we've retired, we are going to sell our house, then buy a boat, then buy a RV, then move to Arizona and buy a house on a golf course and then go to Mexico once a year and play golf and do whatever we want for the rest of our lives."

Chapter 11   Conclusion – Final Thoughts

This is an example of the type of thinking behind a life of the sin of pride, of being self-willed, lawless, out of control and ignoring God's Will for your life. When you truly know His Love for you, when you truly know Him, you can trust Him and not be afraid to give up your life to Him and let Him now be in control of everything. He is a big God, He loves you, He is able to keep you, and He can do a better job of running your lives than you ever could. He created you; He has a plan, a destiny, and a good future for you.

Will you finally "give it up" and just fall into His arms of love and let Him be in charge of everything right now? Will you let go of the "steering wheel" of your life and let Him take the wheel? "Father Knows Best" was the name of a television program when I was a child, will you believe and accept that for you?

As a new Christian, many years ago, I simply made a decision, "I will do everything in this Book (the Bible) that it says to do and not do anything it says not to do." When I did that I put myself in Divine order, I was no longer "out of control" in God's eyes, and God took control. That has worked out well!

Jesus was speaking one day to Nicodemus, a religious leader, He said, "Do not marvel that I said to you, 'You must be born again'. The wind blows where it wishes and you hear the sound of it, but do not know where it comes from and where it is going; so is everyone who is born of the Sprit" (John 3: 7, 8).

Chapter 11   Conclusion – Final Thoughts

When we are "born of the Spirit" and God is no longer just our
Creator but now our "Father," we freely give up control of our own
life and become like a little child following their Daddy! We are like
a leaf in the wind, the wind blows us where it wills, it is in control
and we are not.

This is what Jesus was talking about, He is revealing a revelation to
us, that our life now is like the wind, we don't know "where it is
going" because we are not in control anymore. We have given that
up and now the Spirit of God, the Holy Spirit is leading us into God's
will and destiny for our lives.

God's Word says, *"The Kingdom of God is ... righteousness, peace
and joy in the Holy Spirit"* (Romans 14:17). God desires for you and
me to have peace and joy in our lives. There can be no peace and joy
if we are afraid of getting cancer. When we are in the "Kingdom of
God", living in that Kingdom, we experience "peace and joy" in our
lives, body, soul and spirit. "The Kingdom of God" means God is
ruling as King over His domain, His property, and His subjects.
When He rules over our lives and we subject ourselves to Him as our
King, we enter "The Kingdom of God" and "peace" comes. "Peace"
comes into our body and our cells are at "peace" with us and not out
of control, in disorder, attacking us, and cancer has no place.

Chapter 11   Conclusion – Final Thoughts

Also *"For all who are being led by the Spirit of God, these are the sons of God"* (Romans 8:14). Sons and daughters of God are led by God, they follow, they let the Father lead, they choose out of their own free will to lay down their life and give it over to God to lead as it pleases Him.

This can be real scary and hard to do if we do not know Him or believe He has our best in mind. But He wants us to know Him. He longs for relationship and fellowship. He longs to hear us talk to Him and spend time with Him. He longs as a Good Father to love us and pour down from Heaven *"good things and perfect gifts"* upon us (James 1:17).

Are you ready to make that decision? To cast yourself upon God, to give over complete control to Him and let Him lead and direct your paths? But wait; maybe you are afraid of what will happen if you do that. What are you afraid of? Let's pause a moment and ponder that...!

Are you afraid God will destroy your life? Ruin it? No, of course not, He is your Heavenly Father. He loves you, He made you, and He sent His Son Jesus to give you "abundant life," not ruin your life. He has a plan and a wonderful destiny that will bring you into success and prosperity (Joshua 1:8) if you will let Him.

Chapter 11   Conclusion – Final Thoughts

Maybe you had an earthly father that didn't represent the Heavenly Father's unconditional love and care and protection to you, as he should have. God wants to show you Himself; He is different, and has your best in mind. He wants to shower you with "Good things, Good gifts" (James 1:17). He wants you to trust Him, to fall back into His arms, to let go and let Him take the steering wheel.

Will you change to a unique lifestyle of "Listening and Following" instead of a "Self-Determination and Self-willed" lifestyle?

Talk to God now about this, He understands, He is listening, He is waiting to be your Father, to guide you, help you, bless you and lead you into a successful, prosperous and wonderful destiny.

> *Heavenly Father, I come to you in Jesus Name, I now choose to give up control of my life to you; like Jesus I now say to You, "Not my will, but Your Will be done." Father, fill me with the knowledge of Your will for my life and destiny. You said, 'Follow Me', so Father, I ask you to show me where You are going, what You are doing, what You are saying, what You want to do in any situation. Help me to recognize Your leading, Your Voice, and Your nudging to know the way of this path of life You have planned for me. Forgive me and forgive my family generations for pride, for lawlessness, for being self-willed in our lives. I receive forgiveness now. Thank you Father God, in Jesus Name. Amen!*

Chapter 11   Conclusion – Final Thoughts

If you did that, if you surrendered, if you gave yourself and your life to God, you are ready to enter into that place where your cells in your body are also no longer "out of control," but in "in control" to die when they are to die and live when they are to live.

But first, if you are not yet born-again, but you want to be, you want God your Creator to now be your Father in Heaven, please go to Appendix A, "Will you go to Heaven when you die?" – "How to receive God's Gift of Eternal Life in Heaven," and pray to receive Jesus as your Savior and Lord and be born again.

My prayer for you is that this book has been a blessing to you to help bring you into your God-given destiny and purpose that God put you on this earth to fulfill.

 Please write me with your comments and any questions you may have at:

Richard McIlvaine - P.O. Box 315 , Issaquah, WA USA 98027
Email: RichardMcIlvaine@gmail.com

Appendix A

Will you go to Heaven when you die?
How to receive God's Gift of Eternal Life
in Heaven!

Let's start by hearing God's Plan for your going to Heaven. Please read God's Words from the Bible written below:

"For God so loved the world, that He gave His only begotten Son, that whoever believes in Him shall not perish, but have eternal life.
For God did not send the Son into the world to judge the world, but that the world might be saved through Him.
He who believes in Him is not judged; he who does not believe has been judged already, because he has not believed in the name of the only begotten Son of God." John 3:16-18

Jesus answered, "Truly, truly, I say to you, unless one is born of water and the Spirit he cannot enter into the kingdom of God. That which is born of the flesh is flesh, and that which is born of the Spirit is spirit.
Do not be amazed that I said to you, 'You must be born again.' " John 3:5-7

"For the wages of sin is death, but the free gift of God is eternal life in Christ Jesus
our Lord." Romans 6:23

Who gave you life? God did! Who knows you and wants to remove the guilt from all the things you ever did wrong? God! Who wants to remove all your guilt and sins and remove the fear of death from you? God!

God's Word says, "for all have sinned and fall short of the glory of God,..." Romans 3:23

God has a plan to remove the guilt and sin that separates us from God!

God's Word says, " But God demonstrates His own love toward us, in that while we were yet sinners, Christ died for us." Romans 5:8

Jesus died for you! He suffered our punishment for sin so that we could be with Him forever in Heaven. Jesus loved you that much!

We each need to personally receive what Jesus did for us on the cross in order to receive God's gift of eternal life, be saved, be born again, go to Heaven.

We start by telling God how very sorry we are for the things we did wrong, asking God to forgive us and repenting or turning away from doing wrong things in our life.

God's Word says, "If we confess our sins, He is faithful and righteous to forgive us our sins and to cleanse us from all unrighteousness." 1 John 1:9

And; "Peter {said} to them, 'Repent, and each of you be baptized in the name of Jesus Christ for the forgiveness of your sins; and you will receive the gift of the Holy Spirit.

For the promise is for you and your children and for all who are far off, as many as the Lord our God will call to Himself.' " Acts 2:38,39

And; "But as many as received Him, to them He gave the right to become children of God, {even} to those who believe in His name, who were born, not of blood nor of the will of the flesh nor of the will of man, but of God."   John 1:12,13

Jesus wants you to believe in Him, that He is the Son of God, that He died for you and rose again on the third day and lives today and forever in Heaven with the Father.

God's Word says, "that if you confess with your mouth Jesus {as} Lord, and believe in your heart that God raised Him from the dead, you will be saved; for with the heart a person believes, resulting in righteousness, and with the mouth he confesses, resulting in salvation.
For the Scripture says, "WHOEVER BELIEVES IN HIM WILL NOT BE DISAPPOINTED."   Romans 10: 9-11

What to do to be a child of God, born again, ready to receive His benefits of eternal life, healing, being set free from bondages, peace, wisdom, protection and the list goes on and on.

1.   Ask God to reveal Himself to you! Talk to Him, Ask Him for mercy, for the Holy Spirit to come to you and reveal Jesus and His power.
2.   Confess that you have fallen short of God's plan and sinned and done things wrong and ask for God to forgive you of the things you did wrong.
3.   Be willing to turn away from doing wrong anymore with God's help, this is repenting or turning to go a different way.
4.   Receive Jesus as your personal Savior and believe that He took your sins and your punishment on the cross, died and rose again and lives today and forever.
5.   Finally, pray this prayer or similar from your heart out loud:

"Dear God, I come you in Jesus Name. I believe that Jesus is your Son and that He died on the cross for me and rose again on the third day. I know that I have sinned and need forgiveness. I ask you to forgive me of my sins and wash me clean, free from guilt. I turn away from all wrong and sin and will follow you all the days of my life. I now invite Jesus into my heart and my life and receive Him as my personal Savior and Lord. I receive your free gift of eternal life through what Jesus did on the cross for me. Thank you Heavenly Father in Jesus Name."

What do I do now?

1. Start talking to God daily.

 2. Get a Bible and start reading it every day.

3. Find other Bible believing Christians to fellowship with and pray together with.

4. Find a good Bible believing, Bible teaching, church to go to.

5. Be water baptized.

6. Tell others about Jesus.

7. Start to pray and ask God what His plan is for your life and find your destiny in God.

Appendix B

Scriptures Relating to Generational Curses

Please read and study the following Scriptures to understand more how sin in one generation can and does affect generations following. It is not that God is forcing the sin on the next generation, but the sins of the fathers and mothers are a source of influence, a heavy weight, a pressure, so to speak, for the children to follow in the same sins.

These generational sins being passed down are broken when someone comes to Christ and that generation repents of their sin and becomes free from it. It is usually necessary for others to pray with that person and minister to them in the power of the Holy Spirit to break the power of the past generational sins and influence off their lives and the lives of their children.

God's word in Galatians 5:1 reveals to us, " It was for freedom that Christ set us free; therefore keep standing firm and do not be subject again to a yoke of slavery."

Jesus said, " If therefore the Son shall make you free, you shall be free indeed." John 8:36
Also; "…and you shall know the truth and the truth shall set you free." John 8:32

"Then the LORD said to Cain, 'Where is Abel your brother?' And he said, 'I do not know. Am I my brother's keeper?'
He said, 'What have you done? The voice of your brother's blood is crying to Me from the ground.

Now you are cursed from the ground, which has opened its mouth to receive your brother's blood from your hand.' "   Genesis 4:9-11

"You shall not worship them or serve them; for I, the Lord your God, am a jealous God, visiting the iniquity of the fathers on the children, on the third and the fourth generations of those who hate Me, but showing lovingkindness to thousands, to those who love Me and keep My commandments."   Exodus 20:5-6

"Then the Lord passed by in front of him and proclaimed, 'The Lord, the Lord God, compassionate and gracious, slow to anger, and abounding in lovingkindness and truth;
who keeps lovingkindness for thousands, who forgives iniquity, transgression and sin; yet He will by no means leave {the guilty} unpunished, visiting the iniquity of fathers on the children and on the grandchildren to the third and fourth generations.' "   Exodus 34:6-7

Deuteronomy 5:9 "You shall not worship them or serve them; for I, the LORD your God, am a jealous God, visiting the iniquity of the fathers on the children, and on the third and the fourth {generations} of those who hate Me,
Deut 5:10 but showing lovingkindness to thousands, to those who love Me and keep My commandments."

Numbers 14:33 "Your sons shall be shepherds for forty years in the wilderness, and they will suffer {for} your unfaithfulness, until your corpses lie in the wilderness.
Num 14:34 According to the number of days which you spied out the land, forty days, for every day you shall bear your guilt a year, forty years, and you will know My opposition."

Romans 5:9 "Much more then, having now been justified by His blood, we shall be saved from the wrath {of God} through Him.
Rom 5:10 For if while we were enemies we were reconciled to God through the death of His Son, much more, having been reconciled, we shall be saved by His life."

Romans 7:5 "For while we were in the flesh, the sinful passions, which were {aroused} by the Law, were at work in the members of our body to bear fruit for death.
Rom 7:6 But now we have been released from the Law, having died to that by which we were bound, so that we serve in newness of the Spirit and not in oldness of the letter."

Hebrews 9:22 "And according to the Law, {one may} almost {say,} all things are cleansed with blood, and without shedding of blood there is no forgiveness."

Galatians 5:1 "It was for freedom that Christ set us free; therefore keep standing firm and do not be subject again to a yoke of slavery."

Galatians 3:13 "Christ redeemed us from the curse of the Law, having become a curse for us--for it is written, "CURSED IS EVERYONE WHO HANGS ON A TREE"--
Gal 3:14: in order that in Christ Jesus the blessing of Abraham might come to the Gentiles, so that we would receive the promise of the Spirit through faith."

Appendix C

Scriptures Relating Sin & Sickness Sometimes Tied Together!

Genesis 2:17 "but from the tree of the knowledge of good and evil you shall not eat, for in the day that you eat from it you will surely die."

Deuteronomy 11:26 "See, I am setting before you today a blessing and a curse:
Deut 11:27 the blessing, if you listen to the commandments of the LORD your God, which I am commanding you today;
Deut 11:28 and the curse, if you do not listen to the commandments of the LORD your God, but turn aside from the way which I am commanding you today, by following other gods which you have not known."

Exodus 15:26 "And He said, "If you will give earnest heed to the voice of the LORD your God, and do what is right in His sight, and give ear to His commandments, and keep all His statutes, I will put none of the diseases on you which I have put on the Egyptians; for I, the LORD, am your healer."

Daniel 9:9 "To the Lord our God {belong} compassion and forgiveness, for we have rebelled against Him;
Daniel 9:10 nor have we obeyed the voice of the LORD our God, to walk in His teachings which He set before us through His servants the prophets.
Daniel 9:11 Indeed all Israel has transgressed Your law and turned aside, not obeying Your voice; so the curse has been poured out on us, along with the oath which is written in the law of Moses the servant of God, for we have sinned against Him."

Daniel 9:16 "O Lord, in accordance with all Your righteous acts, let now Your anger and Your wrath turn away from Your city Jerusalem, Your holy mountain; for because of our sins and the
iniquities of our fathers, Jerusalem and Your people {have become} a reproach to all those around us."

Psalm 119:67 "Before I was afflicted I went astray, But now I keep Your word."
Psalm 119:68 "You are good and do good; Teach me Your statutes."

Proverbs 3:7-8 "Do not be wise in your own eyes; Fear the LORD and turn away from evil.
It will be healing to your body and refreshment to your bones."

Matthew 9:5 "Which is easier, to say, 'Your sins are forgiven,' or to say, 'Get up, and walk'?
Matt 9:6 "But so that you may know that the Son of Man has authority on earth to forgive sins"--then He said to the paralytic, "Get up, pick up your bed and go home."

John 5:13 "But the man who was healed did not know who it was, for Jesus had slipped away while there was a crowd in {that} place.
John 5:14 Afterward Jesus found him in the temple and said to him, "Behold, you have become well; do not sin anymore, so that nothing worse happens to you."

John 9:1 "As He passed by, He saw a man blind from birth.

John 9:2 And His disciples asked Him, "Rabbi, <u>who sinned,</u> <u>this man or his parents, that he would be born blind?</u>

John 9:3 Jesus answered, {It was} <u>neither {that} this man</u> <u>sinned, nor his parents; but {it was} so that the works of God might</u> <u>be displayed in him.</u>"

Romans 5:12 "Therefore, just as through one man sin entered into the world, and death through sin, and so death spread to all men, because all sinned."

Romans 6:23 "For the <u>wages of sin is death,</u> but the free gift of God is eternal life in Christ Jesus our Lord."

1 Corinthians 11:29 "For he who eats and drinks, eats and <u>drinks judgment to himself if he does not judge the body rightly.</u>

1 Cor 11:30 For this reason many among you are weak and sick, and a number sleep.

1 Cor 11:31 But <u>if we judged ourselves rightly, we would not</u> <u>be judged.</u>"

Hebrews 12:12-13 "Therefore, strengthen the hands that are weak and the knees that are feeble, and <u>make straight paths for your</u> <u>feet, so that {the limb} which is lame may not be put out of joint, but</u> <u>rather be healed.</u>"

James 5:16 "Therefore, <u>confess your sins to one another, and</u> <u>pray for one another so that you may be healed.</u> The effective prayer of a righteous man can accomplish much."

Appendix D

Scriptures Relating to Sickness Caused by a demonic spirit

Luke 13:11 "And there was a woman who for eighteen years had <u>had a sickness caused by a spirit; and she was bent double</u>, and could not straighten up at all.

Luke 13:12 When Jesus saw her, He called her over and said to her, "Woman, you are freed from your sickness."

Luke 13:13 And He laid His hands on her; and immediately she was made erect again and {began} glorifying God."

Mark 5:1 "They came to the other side of the sea, into the country of the Gerasenes.

Mark 5:2 When He got out of the boat, immediately a man from the tombs with an unclean spirit met Him,

Mark 5:3 and he had his dwelling among the tombs. And no one was able to bind him anymore, even with a chain;

Mark 5:4 because he had often been bound with shackles and chains, and the chains had been torn apart by him and the shackles broken in pieces, and no one was strong enough to subdue him.

Mark 5:5 Constantly, night and day, he was screaming among the tombs and in the mountains, and gashing himself with stones.

Mark 5:6 Seeing Jesus from a distance, he ran up and bowed down before Him;

Mark 5:7 and shouting with a loud voice, he said, "What business do we have with each other, Jesus, Son of the Most High God? I implore You by God, do not torment me!"

Mark 5:8 For He had been saying to him, "Come out of the man, you unclean spirit!"

Mark 5:9 And He was asking him, <u>"What is your name?" And he said to Him, "My name is Legion; for we are many."</u> (<u>example of demons having names</u>)

Mark 5:10 And he {began} to implore Him earnestly not to send them out of the country.

Mark 5:11 Now there was a large herd of swine feeding nearby on the mountain.

Mark 5:12 {The demons} implored Him, saying, "Send us into the swine so that we may enter them."

Mark 5:13 Jesus gave them permission. And coming out, the unclean spirits entered the swine; and the herd rushed down the steep bank into the sea, about two thousand {of them;} and they were drowned in the sea.

Mark 5:15 They came to Jesus and observed the man who had been demon-possessed sitting down, clothed and in his right mind, the very man who had had the "legion"; and they became frightened."

Mark 6:13 "And they were casting out many demons and were anointing with oil many sick people and healing them."

Mark 9:17 "And one of the crowd answered Him, "Teacher, I brought You my son, possessed with a spirit which makes him mute;

Mark 9:18 and whenever it seizes him, it slams him {to the ground} and he foams {at the mouth,} and grinds his teeth and stiffens out. I told Your disciples to cast it out, and they could not {do it.}

Mark 9:19 And He answered them and said, "O unbelieving generation, how long shall I be with you? How long shall I put up with you? Bring him to Me!"

Mark 9:20 They brought the boy to Him. When he saw Him, immediately the spirit threw him into a convulsion, and falling to the ground, he {began} rolling around and foaming {at the mouth.}

Mark 9:21 And He asked his father, "How long has this been happening to him?" And he said, "From childhood.

Mark 9:22 "It has often thrown him both into the fire and into the water to destroy him. But if You can do anything, take pity on us and help us!"

Mark 9:23 And Jesus said to him, " 'If You can?' All things are possible to him who believes."

Mark 9:24 Immediately the boy's father cried out and said, "I do believe; help my unbelief."

Mark 9:25 When Jesus saw that a crowd was rapidly gathering, He rebuked the unclean spirit, saying to it, "You deaf and mute spirit, I command you, come out of him and do not enter him again."

Mark 9:26 After crying out and throwing him into terrible convulsions, it came out; and {the boy} became so much like a corpse that most {of them} said, "He is dead!"

Mark 9:27 But Jesus took him by the hand and raised him; and he got up."

Acts 8:7 "For {in the case of} many who had unclean spirits, they were coming out {of them} shouting with a loud voice; and many who had been paralyzed and lame were healed.

Acts 8:8 So there was much rejoicing in that city."

Acts 16:16 "It happened that as we were going to the place of prayer, a slave-girl having a spirit of divination met us, who was bringing her masters much profit by fortune-telling.

Acts 16:17 Following after Paul and us, she kept crying out, saying, "These men are bond-servants of the Most High God, who are proclaiming to you the way of salvation."

Acts 16:18 She continued doing this for many days. But Paul was greatly annoyed, and turned and said to the spirit, "I command you in the name of Jesus Christ to come out of her!" And it came out at that very moment."

Appendix E

Romans 6: 12-23 relating to lawlessness, "resulting in further lawlessness"- Cancer!

Romans 6:12,13 "Therefore do not let sin reign in your mortal body so that you obey its lusts, and do not go on presenting the members of your body to sin {as} instruments of unrighteousness; but present yourselves to God as those alive from the dead, and your members {as} instruments of righteousness to God."

Rom 6:14 "For sin shall not be master over you, for you are not under law but under grace.

Rom 6:15 What then? Shall we sin because we are not under law but under grace? May it never be!

Rom 6:16 Do you not know that when you present yourselves to someone {as} slaves for obedience, you are slaves of the one whom you obey, either of sin resulting in death, or of obedience resulting in righteousness?

Rom 6:17 But thanks be to God that though you were slaves of sin, you became obedient from the heart to that form of teaching to which you were committed,
Rom 6:18 and having been freed from sin, you became slaves of righteousness.

Rom 6:19 I am speaking in human terms because of the weakness of your flesh. For just as you presented your members as slaves to impurity and to lawlessness, resulting in {further} lawlessness, so now present your members as slaves to righteousness, resulting in sanctification.

Rom 6:20 For when you were slaves of sin, you were free in regard to righteousness.

Rom 6:21 Therefore what benefit were you then deriving from the things of which you are now ashamed? For the outcome of those things is death.

Rom 6:22 But now having been freed from sin and enslaved to God, you derive your benefit, resulting in sanctification, and the outcome, eternal life.

Romans 6:23 For the wages of sin is death, but the free gift of God is eternal life in Christ Jesus our Lord."

Appendix F

Leviathan –crocodile - Job Chapter 41

Job 41:1 "Can you draw out Leviathan with a fishhook? Or press down his tongue with a cord?

Job 41:2 Can you put a rope in his nose or pierce his jaw with a hook?

Job 41:3 Will he make many supplications to you, Or will he speak to you soft words?

Job 41:4 Will he make a covenant with you? Will you take him for a servant forever?

Job 41:5 Will you play with him as with a bird, or will you bind him for your maidens?

Job 41:6 Will the traders bargain over him? Will they divide him among the merchants?

Job 41:7 Can you fill his skin with harpoons, or his head with fishing spears?

Job 41:8 Lay your hand on him; Remember the battle; you will not do it again!

Job 41:9 Behold, your expectation is false; Will you be laid low even at the sight of him?

Job 41:10 No one is so fierce that he dares to arouse him; Who then is he that can stand before Me?

Job 41:11 Who has given to Me that I should repay {him?} {Whatever} is under the whole heaven is Mine.

Job 41:12 I will not keep silence concerning his limbs, Or his mighty strength, or his orderly frame.

Job 41:13 Who can strip off his outer armor? Who can come within his double mail?

Job 41:14 Who can open the doors of his face? Around his teeth there is terror.

Job 41:15 {His} strong scales are {his} pride, Shut up {as with} a tight seal.

Job 41:16 One is so near to another that no air can come between them.

Job 41:17 They are joined one to another; They clasp each other and cannot be separated.

Job 41:18 His sneezes flash forth light, And his eyes are like the eyelids of the morning.

Job 41:19 Out of his mouth go burning torches; Sparks of fire leap forth.

Job 41:20 Out of his nostrils smoke goes forth As {from} a boiling pot and {burning} rushes.

Job 41:21 His breath kindles coals, And a flame goes forth from his mouth.

Job 41:22 In his neck lodges strength, And dismay leaps before him.

Job 41:23 The folds of his flesh are joined together, Firm on him and immovable.

Job 41:24 His heart is as hard as a stone, even as hard as a lower millstone.

Job 41:25 When he raises himself up, the mighty fear; Because of the crashing they are bewildered.

Job 41:26 The sword that reaches him cannot avail, nor the spear, the dart or the javelin.

Job 41:27 He regards iron as straw, Bronze as rotten wood.

Job 41:28 The arrow cannot make him flee; Slingstones are turned into stubble for him.

Job 41:29 Clubs are regarded as stubble; He laughs at the rattling of the javelin.

Job 41:30 His underparts are {like} sharp potsherds; He spreads out {like} a threshing sledge on the mire.

Job 41:31 He makes the depths boil like a pot; He makes the sea like a jar of ointment.

Job 41:32 Behind him he makes a wake to shine; one would think the deep to be gray-haired.

Job 41:33 Nothing on earth is like him, One made without fear.

Job 41:34 **He looks on (to attack) everything that is high; (where there is pride)**

      He is king (does whatever he wants to steal, kill, and destroy) over all the sons of pride."

Recommended Resources List

Books / Booklets / Tapes / Cd's / Information

"The Bible" – see all verses on healing   order information: any Christian bookstore, Amazon.com , other stores

"Healing Belongs to Us" – Kenneth E. Hagin   small booklet / cassette series
    order information: Kenneth Hagin Ministries P.O. Box 50126, Tulsa,OK 74150
    or telephone 1 888-28-faith or website: www.rhema.org
    (see many other books/tapes/videos on healing from this ministry)

"Jesus the Healer" – E.W. Kenyon (booklet or 2 tape audio tape series)
    order from: Kenyon's Gospel Publishing Society, P.O. Box 973, Lynnwood,WA 98046
    website: www.kenyons.org

"Active or Passive Lordship" by Fred Markert, "Article-4 pages", Last Days Ministries
    order from: website: www.lastdaysministries.org

"How to Live and Not Die" by Norvel Hayes book   or 6 part cassette series
Norvel Hayes Ministries - Telephone: 423-479-5434   website: www.nhm.cc
New Life Bible Church - 155 S. Ocoee St . Cleveland , TN 37311

"Humility"; the hidden power of Humility" by John Bevere (2 part CD series)
order information: John Bevere Ministries, website : www.johnbevere.org
Telephone: 1 800 648-1477
("Humility strengthens and protects you from the enemy. It keeps you sensitive to the heart of God so He can reveal His ways...and it empowers us to complete the race. In Psalms 25:9 we learn God...leads the humble in what is right, teaching them His way. Humility is a characteristic of His nature we are to excel in." - John Bevere)

"Humility vs. Pride"   Chart by Joy Dawson
Source & permission to use pending contact/permission from Joy Dawson –Teacher / YWAM

About the Writer

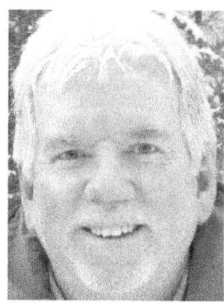

Rev. Richard K. McIlvaine

President- New Life Christian Fellowship, Inc.

Author: "Cancer Healing" , "Seven Keys to Prevent Cancer"
"The Father's Face",   "Enter My Rest" ,
"The Father's Face"   in Korean and English,
" Enter My Rest"   in Korean and English

Present Ministry: Traveling Ministry - Conferences - Churches
- Bible Schools - Discipleship

Richard & Joy McIlvaine have served in ministry for over 31
years in a variety of different areas.

Richard has served as a Royal Rangers leader, Sunday school
teacher, a church elder, Bible school teacher, Licensed in 1983,
Ordained in 1985, Senior Pastor of New Life Christian
Fellowship, Inc. for 7 years, traveling ministry locally and
abroad since 1991, Bible School director, Short term
Missionary in South Korea doing a Bible School for 75 Korean
pastors in 1998, and Founder/Director of the Divine Healing
Rooms - Seattle Eastside ministry along with his wife Joy for 8
years until April of 2008, to return to more full time traveling
ministry and writing.

Richard & Joy continue to travel locally and overseas to bring encouragement and healing to the Body of Christ. Their ministry has a prophetic aspect to it and they seek to listen to the Holy Spirit and bring fresh teaching, impartation, personal ministry, and healing the sick to those they minister to. They also continue to oversee " New Life Christian Fellowship, Inc." a fellowship of churches, ministers and intercessors in ministry and missions that also gives Licensing and Ordination those called into ministry.

Richard was saved in 1977 while working for Continental Airlines in Seattle, WA. A number of Christians witnessed and shared the gospel with him. But it was a message given one day on television through the "700 Club" program with Pat Robertson that resulted in him being born-again. Previous to that time he had been brought up in the Catholic church and later attended and graduated from St. Joseph's High School, St. Croix, U.S. Virgin Islands.

A year after being saved, he began attending "Faith Tabernacle" church, Kent, WA, a full-gospel church associated with the (FCA) "Fellowship of Christian Assemblies" a group similar to the "Assemblies of God" churches, but non-denominational. He later graduated from "Faith Bible Training Center" after 2 years of studying God's Word and doing internship work in their Christian school "Faith Academy". It was there that Pastor Richard Martin taught him a deep love for the Word of God and to preach the Word of God expecting it to produce fruit in people's lives. Shortly later he became one of the elders of New Life Christian Fellowship, Issaquah,WA and shortly later appointed Senior Pastors of New Life Christian Fellowship and pastored there for seven years before going into traveling ministry.

Richard & Joy have been married for 31 years and have three wonderful children, Anna, John and David.

They reside in the beautiful Seattle- Eastside area of the Pacific Northwest and enjoy the beauty and activities available to the area.

They continue to minister locally and travel internationally to minister as the Lord leads them.

Richard continues to minister in South Korea frequently in churches and Bible schools, and YWAM bases, etc.

 Richard also enjoys family time, photography, and hiking, writing.

Joy presently serves on staff at Seattle Revival Center, Newcastle, WA in children's ministry.

****
****

Richard McIlvaine can be contacted at :

P.O. Box 315 - ISSAQUAH , WA USA 98027

RichardMcIlvaine@gmail.com

Cancer Healing   Richard K McIlvaine

Book - "Cancer Healing"

Disclaimer for Book, Prayers or Ministry offered!

Please note that this Book presents ministering materials to people based on teaching and believing God's Word in the Bible and healing prayer in Jesus' Name and is intended primarily, but not exclusively, for born again Christians seeking to receive spiritual healing from God.)

The book "Cancer Healing", in no way claims to guarantee a cure or healing of any disease, sickness, illness, condition, or cancer.

Due to possible varying results obtained by individuals reading and applying the book "Cancer Healing" being not in our hands but in the "Hands of God", Who is the One presented as healing people and not us, we do not claim to be able to heal or cure anyone of cancer or illness.
The Book presents materials, teaching, and prayer that involves unknown factors that could possibly affect the results an individual may experience.

The results an individual may possibly experience involve factors that are not in the above book such as God's Will, the mercy of God, other unknown factors present in the person's life, the individual persons heart response to the will of God, the teaching, or the prayer to God offered.

We are not doctors and as such do not prescribe medicine nor can advise a person to take or not take medicine, start or stop medical care.
The submitting of gifts, book donations, donations, etc. in no way guarantee's a person's receiving healing or a cure of illness or cancer.

Any donations received are used to support the ministry and reflect not only the expenses of the ministry but the support of the overall vision and mission of the ministry and its international outreaches.

Disclaimer Presented by: Rev. Richard and Joy McIlvaine and New Life Christian Fellowship, Inc. Issaquah, WA USA.

www.ingramcontent.com/pod-product-compliance
Lightning Source LLC
Chambersburg PA
CBHW060522290526
45791CB00001B/501